SURGICAL RECALL

SURGICAL RECALL

SENIOR EDITOR

Lorne H. Blackbourne, M.D.

Resident in General Surgery
Department of Surgery
University of Virginia
Charlottesville, Virginia

EDITORS

John Minasi, M.D.

Assistant Professor
Department of Surgery
Division of General Surgery
University of Virginia
Charlottesville, Virginia

Douglas Newburg, Ph.D.

Director of Performance Education
Department of Surgery
University of Virginia
Charlottesville, Virginia

Curtis G. Tribble, M.D.

Associate Professor
Department of Surgery
Division of Thoracic-Cardiovascular Surgery
University of Virginia
Charlottesville, Virginia

Williams & Wilkins

BALTIMORE • PHILADELPHIA • HONG KONG
LONDON • MUNICH • SYDNEY • TOKYO

A WAVERLY COMPANY

Editor: Timothy S. Satterfield
Managing Editor: Linda S. Napora
Copy Editor: Anne K. Schwartz
Designer: Wilma E. Rosenberger
Illustration Planner: Lorraine Wrzosek
Production Coordinator: Anne Stewart Seitz

Copyright © 1994
Williams & Wilkins
428 East Preston Street
Baltimore, Maryland 21202, USA

Printed in the United States of America

Library of Congress Cataloging in Publication Data

Surgical recall / senior editor, Lorne H. Blackbourne, editors, John
  Minasi, Doug Newburg, Curtis G. Tribble.
      p. cm.
    Includes index.
    ISBN 0-683-00835-8
    1. Surgery—Examinations, questions, etc.   I. Blackbourne, Lorne
  H.
    [DNLM: 1. Surgery, Operative—examination questions.   WO 18 S9615
  1994]
  RD37.2.S9748   1994
  617′.0076—dc20
  DNLM/DLC
  for Library of Congress   94-5559
                                                                CIP

                                                        96   97   98
                                       3   4   5   6   7   8   9   10

CONTRIBUTORS

The following contributed to this book while they were medical students at the University of Virginia Health Sciences Center:

1989—Lorne H. Blackbourne, M.D.

1990—Lorne H. Blackbourne, M.D.

1991—Kirk J. Fleischer, M.D.
Colt Peyton, M.D.

1992—Oliver A. R. Binns, M.D.
Christopher Bogaev, M.D.
R. Bradford Bowles III, M.D.
James A. Burns, M.D.
David deHoll, M.D.
Hong J. Kim, M.D.
Carolyn Lederman, M.D.
L. Carr McClain, M.D.
Gregory Paine, M.D.
Richard S. Polin, M.D.
Henry M. Prillaman, M.D.
Donald Schmidt, M.D.
Walter Scott, M.D.
Nathan E. Simmons, M.D.
Owen B. Tabor, M.D.
Anne Whitworth, M.D.

1993—Linda C. Ahn, M.D.
Robert A. Buckmire, M.D.
David C. Cassada, M.D.
John W. Davis, M.D.
Nicolisa DeSouza, M.D.
Barbara M. Fried, M.D.
W. Glover Garner, M.D.
Christopher Hogan, M.D.
Nancy A. Huff, M.D.
Stephen S. Kim, M.D.
Timothy Kwiatkowski, M.D.
J. Pieter Noordzij, M.D.
David M. Powell, M.D.
G. Bino Rucker, M.D.
Julius P. Smith III, M.D.
Mehrdad Soroush, M.D.
John Sperling, M.D.
Sandeep S. Teja, M.D.
Eric E. Walk, M.D.
T. Lisle Whitman, M.D.
William J. Wirostko, M.D.

REVIEWERS

The following Attending Surgeons and Surgical Residents at the University of Virginia reviewed the material in this book:

Joseph Bianchi, M.D.
Scott A. Buchanan, M.D.
Eugene F. Foley, M.D.
Thomas Gampper, M.D.
John B. Hanks, M.D.
R. Scott Jones, M.D.
Irving L. Kron, M.D.

Scott E. Langenburg, M.D.
Michael C. Mauney, M.D.
Timothy L. Pruett, M.D.
James Reibel, M.D.
W. S. Schenk, M.D.
Craig Slingluff, M.D.

This manual is dedicated to the memory of Leslie E. Rudolf, Professor of Surgery and Vice-Chairman of the Department of Surgery. Dr. Rudolf was born on November 12, 1927 in New Rochelle, New York. He served in the U.S. Army Counter-intelligence Corps after World War II in Europe. He graduated from Union College in 1951 and attended Cornell Medical College where he graduated in 1955. He then entered his surgical residency at Peter Brent Brigham Hospital in Boston, Massachusetts and completed his residency there serving as Chief Resident Surgeon in 1961.

Dr. Rudolf came to Charlottesville, Virginia, as an Assistant Professor of Surgery in 1963. He rapidly rose through the ranks, becoming Professor of Surgery and Vice-Chairman of the Department in 1974 and a Markle Scholar in Academic Medicine from 1966 until 1971. His research interests included organ and tissue transplantation and preservation. Dr. Rudolf was instrumental in initiating the Kidney Transplant Program at the University of Virginia Health Sciences Center. His active involvement in service to the Charlottesville community is particularly exemplified by his early work with the Charlottesville/Albemarle Rescue Squad, and received the Governor's Citation for the Commonwealth of Virginia Emergency Medical Services in 1980.

His colleagues at the University of Virginia Health Sciences Center, including faculty and residents, recognized his keen interests in teaching medical students, evaluation and teaching of residents, and his interest in the young surgical faculty. He took a serious interest in medical student education, and he would have strongly approved of this teaching manual, affectionately known as the "Rudolf" guide, as an extension of ward rounds and textbook reading.

In addition to Dr. Rudolf's distinguished academic accomplishments, he was a talented person with many diverse scholarly pursuits and hobbies. His advice and counsel on topics ranging from Chinese cooking to orchid raising was sought by a wide spectrum of friends and admirers.

This manual is a logical extension of Dr. Rudolf's interest in teaching. No one book, operation, or set of rounds can begin to answer all questions of surgical disease processes; however, in a constellation of learning endeavors, this effort would certainly have pleased him.

John B. Hanks, M.D.
Professor of Surgery
University of Virginia
Charlottesville, Virginia

Foreword

Surgical Recall represents the combination of several years' effort by Lorne Blackbourne and his friends who began the project when they were third year medical students. Lorne, now a senior assistant resident in the Department of Surgery, has involved other surgical residents and medical students to provide annual updates and revisions. This reflects the interest, enthusiasm, and true dedication to learning and teaching that permeates the medical school classes and the surgical residencies in our institution. It is an honor, a privilege, and a continuing stimulus to work in the midst of this group of dedicated young people. I congratulate all of the students and residents involved in this project and also acknowledge the leadership of the surgical faculty. The professor's ultimate satisfaction occurs when all the learners assume ownership of learning and teaching.

This book encompasses the essential information in General Surgery and the Surgical Specialties usually imparted to students in our surgical clerkship and reviewed and developed further in electives. Developed from the learner's standpoint the text includes fundamental information such as a description of the diseases, signs, symptoms, essentials of pathophysiology, treatments, and possible outcomes. The unique format of this study guide exploits the Socratic method by employing a list of questions or problems posed along the left side of the page with answers and responses on the right. In addition, the guide includes numerous practical tips to student and junior residents to facilitate comprehensive and effective management of patients. This material is essential for students in the core course of surgery and for those taking senior electives.

We hope you find this guide stimulating and easy to use. We welcome your comments and suggestions.

R. Scott Jones, M.D.
Professor and Chairman
Department of Surgery
University of Virginia
Charlottesville, Virginia

Preface

Surgical Recall began as a source of surgical facts when I was a third and fourth year medical student. Since that time other medical students at the University of Virginia have helped with revisions and additional chapters. Our goal has been to provide concise information that every third year surgical clerk should know.

The format of *Surgical Recall* is conducive to the recall of basic surgical facts because it relies upon repetition and positive feedback. As one repeats the question and answer format, one gains success.

We have dedicated our work to the living memory of Professor Leslie Rudolf.

Lorne H. Blackbourne, M.D.
Resident in General Surgery
University of Virginia
Charlottesville, Virginia

Contents

SECTION *III*   **Subspecialty Surgery**

SECTION *I*

Overview and Background Information

1
Introduction

This study guide was written to accompany the surgical clerkship. It has evolved over the years through student feedback and continued updating. In this regard we welcome any feedback (both positive and negative) or suggestions for improvement. The objective of the guide is to provide a rapid overview of common surgical topics, but keep in mind that it **is NOT written as an all-encompassing source (i.e., you will have to consult major textbooks to round out the information in this guide). The guide is organized in a self-study/quiz format. BY COVERING THE INFORMATION/ANSWERS ON THE RIGHT WITH THE BOOKMARK, YOU CAN ATTEMPT TO ANSWER THE QUESTIONS ON THE LEFT TO ASSESS YOUR UNDERSTANDING OF THE INFORMATION. Keep the guide with you at all times, and when you get even a few minutes (e.g., between cases) hammer out a page or at least a few questions.**

Studying for the Surgery Clerkship

Your study objectives in surgery should include the following 4 points:

1. **OR question and answer periods**
2. **Ward questioning**
3. **Oral exam**
4. **Written exam**

The optimal plan of action would include daily reading in a text such as the Lawrence text, anatomy review prior to each OR case, and this guide—but remember, this guide helps you recall basic facts about surgical topics. Reading should be done daily! The average general surgery clerkship is 6 weeks or 42 days. ** If you read 10 pages a day, that is 420 pages or the entire Lawrence text! As you read the text, take notes.

Granted it is hard to read after a full day in the OR. For a change go to sleep right away and wake up a few hours early the next day and read **before** going to the hospital. It sounds crazy but it does work.

Presenting on Rounds

Your presentation on rounds should be like an iceberg. State important points about your patient (the iceberg visible above the ocean), but know **everything** else about your patient that your Chief might ask about (the iceberg under the ocean). Always include

1. Name
2. Postop day s/p—Procedure
3. Vital signs/temp status/abx day
   Change in physical exam
4. Output—urine/drains
5. Any complaints (not yours—the patient's)
6. Plan

Your presentation should be concise, with good eye contact (you should not simply read from a clipboard). One cannot overemphasize the intangible element of confidence—but if you do not know the answer to a question about a patient the correct response should be "I do not know, but I will find out." Never lie or hedge on an answer to a question; this will only serve to make the remainder of your surgical rotation less than desirable. Furthermore, do your best to be enthusiastic and motivated. **Never, ever whine.** And remember to be a **team player**—never make your fellow students look bad! Residents pick up on this immediately and will slam you.

Operating Room

Your job in the OR will be to retract (water-skiing) and answer questions posed by the attending and residents. Retracting is basically idiot-proof. Many put emphasis on anticipating the surgeons' next move, but as a student stick to following the surgeon's request. Over 75% of the questions asked in the OR deal with anatomy; therefore read about the anatomy and pathophysiology of the case, which will reduce the "I don't knows." Never argue with the scrub nurse—they are always right. They are the selfless warriors of the operating suite's sterile field, and arguing with one will only **make matters worse.**

SURGICAL NOTES

History and Physical Report

The history and physical exam report, better known as the H&P, can make the difference between life and death, and you should take this responsibility very **seriously.** Fatal errors can be made in the H&P, including the incorrect diagnosis, the wrong medications, the wrong allergies, and the wrong PSH. Operative reports of the patient's past surgical procedures are worth their weight in gold! The surgical H&P needs to be both accurate and **concise.** To save space, use − for a negative sign/Sx and + for a positive sign/Sx.

Example H&P (very brief—for illustrative purposes only):

Mr. Smith is a 22 y.o. white male who was in his normal state of excellent health until he noted the onset of periumbilical pain one day prior to admission. This pain was followed approximately 4 hours later by pain located in his right lower quadrant. This pain is exacerbated by any movement. + vomiting, anorexia.

− fever, urinary tract Sx, change in bowel habits, constipation, BRBPR, hematem-
esis, or diarrhea.

Medications: ibuprofen prn headaches
Allergies: NKDA (no known drug allergies)
PMH: none
PSH: none
ROS: − resp dz, − cardiac dz, − renal dz
PE:

heent	ncat, tms clear
cor	nsr, −m,r,g
pulm	clear b/l
abd	nondistended, +bs, +tender RLQ, +rebound RLQ
rectal	guaiac −, nl tone, − mass
ext	nt, −c,c,e
neuro	wnl

LABS: urinalysis (ua) negative. chem 7, PT/PTT, CBC pending
XRAYS: none
ASSESSMENT: 22 y.o. wm with hx and physical findings of right lower quad-
rant peritoneal signs consistent with (c/w) appendicitis.
Plan:
  Consent
  IVF with lactated Ringer's
  IV cefoxitin
  To OR for appendectomy

Wilson Tyler cc III/

Preop Note

The preop note is written in the progress notes the day before the operation.

Example:		
	Preop Dx:	Colon CA
	Labs:	CBC, CHEM 7, PT/PTT
	CXR:	− infiltrate
	Blood:	T & C × 2 units
	ECG:	NSR, wnl
	Anesthesia:	Pre-op completed
	Consent:	Signed and on front of chart
	Orders:	1. Void OCTOR (on call to OR)
		2. 1 gm cefoxitin OCTOR
		3. Hibiclens scrub this p.m.
		4. Bowel prep today
		5. NPO P midnight (MN)

Op Note

The op note is written in the OR before the patient is in the PACU (or recovery
room) in the progress note section of the chart.

Example:

Preop Dx:	Appendicitis
Postop Dx:	Same
Procedure:	Appendectomy
Surgeons:	Halsted
Assistants:	Cushing, Johns cc III
Op findings:	No perforation
Anesthesia:	GET (general endotracheal)
I/O:	1000 ml LR/ uo 600 ml
EBL:	50 ml
Specimen:	Appendix to pathology
Drains:	None
Complications:	None (if there are complications **ask** what you should write)

To PACU in stable condition (PACU = postanesthesia care unit)
cc III = clinical clerk, third year
EBL = estimated blood loss
I/O = Ins and outs

Postop Note

The postop note is written on the day of the operation in the progress notes.

Example:

Procedure:	Appendectomy
Neuro:	A and O $\times$ 3
V/S:	Stable/afebrile
I/O:	1 L LR/ uop 600 ml (urine output)
Labs:	post-op Hct: 36
PE:	cor RRR
	pulm CTA
	abd drsg dry & intact
Drains:	JP 30 ml serosanguinous fluid
Assess:	Stable postop
Plan:	1. IV hydration
	2. 1 gm cefoxitin q 8 hr

Admission Orders

The admission orders are written in the physician orders section of the patient's chart on admission, transfer, or postop.

Example: Admit to 5E Dr. DeBakey

Dx:	AAA
Condition:	Guarded, stable, critical
V/S:	q 4 hr or q shift
	if post-op, q 15 min $\times$ 2 hr, then q 1 hr
	$\times$ 4, then q 4 hr
Activity:	Bedrest or OOB to chair (OOB = out of bed)

Nursing: Daily wgt, I/O
                Drsg-wet to dry q shift
                Call HO for: Temp >38.5
                               UO < 30 ml/hr
                               SBP > 180 < 90
                               DBP >100
                               HR <60 >110

Diet:
IVF:
Drugs:
Labs:

HO = House Officer

Daily Note—Progress Note

Basically an S.O.A.P. note, but one need not write out S.O.A.P. For many reasons, make your notes very objective and do not mention discharge, as this leads to confusion.

Example: 10/1/90 Blue Surgery
                  POD #4 s/p appendectomy
                  Day #5 cefoxitin
                  Pt without c/o
                  V/S: 120/80 76 12 afebrile (Tmax 38)
                  I/O: 1000/600
                  Drains: JP #1 60 last shift (JP = Jackson-Pratt drain)
                  PE: cor   RRR-no m,g,r
                        pulm   CTA
                        abd   +BS, +flatus, −rigidity
                        ext   nt, −cyanosis, −erythema
                               (nt = nontender)

                  ASSESS: Stable POD #4 on IV abx
                  PLAN: 1. Increase PO intake
                         2. Increase ambulation
                         3. Follow cultures

                                               J. Bleau, cc III/

** Always sign your notes and leave room for them to be cosigned!

POD = Postop day (The day after operation is POD 1. The day of operation is the operative day. **But note: antibiotic day #1 is the day the antibiotics were started.)

The acronym for what one should check on your patient daily before rounding with the surgical team: AVOID WTE

A Appearance—any subjective complaints
V Vital signs
O Output—urine/drains

I   Intake—IV/PO
D   Drains—# of/output/character
W   Wound/dressing/weight
T   Temperature
E   Exam—cor, pulm, abd, etc.

COMMON ABBREVIATIONS YOU SHOULD KNOW _____

ā	Before
AAA	Abdominal aortic aneurysm
ABG	Arterial blood gas
AKA	Above the knee amputation
A.K.A.	Also known as
APR	Abdominoperineal resection
ARDS	Adult respiratory distress syndrome
ASA	Aspirin
Ao	Aorta
AXR	Abdominal x-ray
BCP	Birth control pill
BKA	Below the knee amputation
BS	Bowel sounds
BRBPR	Bright red blood per rectum
C̄	With
CA	Cancer
CVA	Cerebral vascular accident
CP	Chest pain
CXR	Chest x-ray
CABG	Coronary artery bypass graft ("CABBAGE")
COPD	Chronic obstructive pulmonary disease
CVP	Central venous pressure
Dx	Diagnosis
DI	Diabetes insipidus
DDx	Differential diagnosis
EBL	Estimated blood loss
EGD	Endoscopic gastroduodenoscopy (UGI scope)
ERCP	Endoscopic retrograde cholangiopancreatography
ETOH	Alcohol
FNA	Fine needle aspiration
GU	Genitourinary
HO	House officer
IABP	Intra-aortic balloon pump
IBD	Inflammatory bowel disease
I&D	Incision and drainage
IVC	Inferior vena cava
IVF	Intravenous fluids
IVP	Intravenous pyelography
IVPB	Intravenous piggyback
L	Left

LAP APPY	Laparoscopic appendectomy
LAP CHOLE	Laparoscopic cholecystectomy
LE	Lower extremity
LES	Lower esophageal sphincter
LR	Lactated Ringer's
LUQ	Left upper quadrant
LLQ	Left lower quadrant
MEN	Multiple endocrine neoplasia
MI	Myocardial infarction
MSO$_4$	Morphine sulfate
NGT	Nasogastric tube
NPO	Nothing per os
NS	Normal saline
OOB	Out of bed
OCTOR	On call to OR
PCWP	Pulmonary capillary wedge pressure
P̄	After
PE	Pulmonary embolism
PEG	Percutaneous endoscopic gastrostomy (via EGD and skin incision)
PGV	Proximal gastric vagotomy, i.e., leaves fibers to pylorus intact to preserve emptying
PID	Pelvic inflammatory disease
PO	Per os (by mouth)
PR	Per rectum
PRN	As needed
PTC	Percutaneous transhepatic cholangiogram (dye injected via a catheter through skin and into dilated intrahepatic bile duct)
PTCA	Percutaneous transluminal coronary angioplasty
PTX	pneumothorax
q̄	Every
QD	Every day
QOD	Every other day
R	Right
Rx	Treatment
RTC	Return to clinic
SBO	Small bowel obstruction
SIADH	Syndrome of inappropriate antidiuretic hormone
SVC	Superior vena cava
S̄	Without
Sx	Symptoms
TEE	Transesophageal echocardiography
T&C	Type and cross
T&S	Type and screen
TPN	Total parenteral nutrition
TURP	Transurethral resection of the prostate
UGI	Upper gastrointestinal
UO	Urine output

US	Ultrasound
UE	Upper extremity
UTI	Urinary tract infection
W→D	Wet to dry dressing
XRT	X-ray therapy
ZE	Zollinger-Ellison syndrome
−	No, negative
+	Yes, positive
↑	Increase, more
↓	Decrease, less
<	Less than
>	Greater than

GLOSSARY OF SURGICAL TERMS YOU SHOULD KNOW

Ablation	The removal of tissue
Abscess	Localized collection of pus anywhere in the body, surrounded and walled off by damaged and inflamed tissues
Achalasia	Condition in which normal muscular activity of the esophagus is decreased, with decreased relaxation of the LES, delaying the passage of swallowed material
Achlorhydria	Absence of hydrochloric acid in the stomach
Acholic stool	Light-colored stool, due to a decreased bile content
Acro-	Prefix denoting extremity or tip
Acronym	Word formed from the initial letter of words
Adeno-	Prefix denoting gland or glands
Adhesion	Union of two normally separate surfaces
Adnexa	Adjoining parts; usually means ovary/fallopian tube
Adventitia	Outer coat of the wall of a vein or artery (composed of loose connective tissue)
Afferent	Toward
-algia	Suffix denoting pain
Amaurosis fugax	Transient visual loss in one eye
Ampulla	Enlarged or dilated ending of a tube or canal
Analgesic	Drug that prevents pain
Anastomosis	Connection between two tubular organs or parts

Anergy	Lack of response to a specific antigen
Angio-	Prefix denoting blood or lymph vessels
Anomaly	Any deviation from the normal i.e. congenital or developmental defect
Apnea	Cessation of breathing
Atelectasis	Failure of the lung to expand/collapse of alveoli
Bariatric	Weight reduction; bariatric surgery is performed on the morbidly obese to effect weight loss
Bezoar	Mass of swallowed foreign material within the stomach
Bifurcation	Point at which division into two branches occurs
Bile salts	Alkaline salts of bile necessary for the emulsification of fats
Bili-	Prefix denoting bile
-blast	Suffix denoting a formative cell type
Blepharo-	Prefix denoting eyelid
Boil	Tender inflamed area of the skin containing pus
Bovie	Electrocautery
Cachexia	Condition of abnormally low weight associated with chronic disease
Calculus	Stone
Calor	Heat, one of the classic signs of inflammation
Cannula	Hollow tube designed for insertion into a body cavity or blood vessel
Carbuncle	A collection of boils (furuncle) with multiple drainage channels (**CAR**buncle = car = big)
Caseation	Breakdown of diseased tissue into a cheese-like material
Caudal	Relating to the lower part or tail of the body
Cauterization	Destruction of tissue by direct application of heat
Cecostomy	Operation in which the cecum is brought to the abdominal wall and opened to decompress or drain the large intestine via a tube
-cele (coele)	Suffix denoting swelling, hernia, or tumor
Celi-	Prefix denoting the abdomen

Celiotomy	Surgical incision into the peritoneal cavity (laparotomy = celiotomy)
Cephal-	Prefix denoting the head
Chole-	Prefix denoting bile
Cholecyst-	Prefix denoting gallbladder
Choledocho-	Prefix denoting the common bile duct
Chyme	Semiliquid acid mass of food that passes from the stomach to the duodenum
Cicatrix	Scar
Cleido-	Prefix denoting the clavicle
Colic	Intermittent abdominal pain indicating pathology in a tubular organ (e.g., small bowel)
Colonoscopy	Endoscopic examination of the colon
Colostomy	Surgical operation in which part of the colon is brought through the abdominal wall to drain or decompress the intestine
Constipation	Infrequent or difficult passage of stool
Cor pulmonale	Enlargement of the right ventricle caused by lung disease and resultant pulmonary hypertension
Curettage	Scraping of the internal surface of an organ or body cavity by means of a spoon-shaped instrument
Cyst	Abnormal sac or closed cavity lined with epithelium and filled with fluid or semisolid material
Direct bilirubin	Conjugated bilirubin (*in*direct = *un*conjugated)
Dolor	Pain, one of the classic signs of inflammation
-dynia	Suffix denoting pain
Dys-	Prefix: difficult/painful/abnormal
Dysphagia	Difficulty in swallowing
Dyspareunia	Painful sexual intercourse
Ecchymosis	Bruise
-ectomy	Suffix denoting the surgical removal of a part or all of an organ (e.g., gastrectomy)
Efferent	Away from

Endarterectomy	Surgical removal of an atheroma and the inner part of the vessel wall to relieve an obstruction (carotid endarterectomy = CEA)
Enteritis	Inflammation of the small intestine, usually causing diarrhea
Enterolysis	Lysis of peritoneal adhesions; not to be confused with enteroclysis, which is a contrast study of the small bowel
Eschar	Scab produced by the action of heat or a corrosive substance on the skin
Excisional biopsy	Biopsy with removal of entire tumor
Falciform ligament	Fold of peritoneum attaching liver to the diaphragm and the anterior abdominal wall as far caudal as the umbilicus; it also contains the ligamentum teres (the obliterated umbilical vein)
Fascia	Sheet of connective tissue
Fistula	Abnormal communication between two hollow, epithelialized organs or between a hollow organ and the exterior (skin)
Foley	Bladder catheter
Frequency	Abnormally increased frequency (e.g., urinary frequency)
Furuncle	Boil, small subcutaneous staphylococcal infection of follicle (think *f*uruncle = *f*ollicle < *c*ar = *c*arbuncle)
Gastropexy	Surgical attachment of the stomach to the abdominal wall
Hemangioma	Benign tumor of blood vessels
Hematemesis	Vomiting of blood
Hematoma	Accumulation of blood within the tissues, which clots to form a solid swelling
Hemoptysis	Coughing up blood
Hemothorax	Blood in the pleural cavity
Hepato-	Prefix denoting the liver
Herniorrhaphy	Surgical repair of a hernia
Hesitancy	Difficulty in initiating urination
Hiatus	Opening or aperture

Hidradenitis	Inflammation of the sweat glands, usually caused by blockage of the glands
Icterus	Jaundice
Ileus	Abnormal intestinal motility (usually paralytic)
Ileostomy	Surgical connection between the lumen of the ileum and the skin of the abdominal wall
Incisional biopsy	Biopsy with only a "slice" of tumor removed
Induration	Abnormal hardening of a tissue or organ
Intussusception	Telescoping of one part of the bowel into another
-itis	Suffix denoting inflammation of an organ, tissue, etc. (e.g., gastritis)
Laparotomy	Surgical incision into the abdominal cavity (laparotomy = celiotomy)
Laparoscopy	Visualization of the peritoneal cavity via a laparoscope
Lap appy	Appendectomy via laparoscopy
Lap chole	Cholecystectomy via laparoscopy
Leiomyoma	Benign tumor of smooth muscle
Leiomyosarcoma	Malignant tumor of smooth muscle
Lieno-	Prefix denoting spleen
-lith	Suffix denoting calculus
Melena	Black tarry feces due to the presence of partly digested blood; occurs when >100 ml (approx.) of blood has entered the gut
Necrotic	Dead
Obstipation	Failure to pass flatus or stool
Odynophagia	Painful swallowing
Onco-	Prefix denoting tumor
Orchi-	Prefix denoting the testes
-orraphy	Surgical repair (e.g., herniorraphy)
-ostomy	General term referring to any operation in which an artificial opening is created between two hollow organs or between one viscera and the abdominal wall for drainage purposes (e.g., colostomy) or for feeding (e.g., gastrostomy)

-otomy   Suffix denoting surgical incision into an organ

Percutaneous   Performed through the skin

-pexy   Suffix denoting fixation

Phleb-   Prefix denoting vein or relating to veins

Phlebolith   Concretion in a vein

Phlegmon   Solid, swollen, inflamed mass of pancreatic tissue

Plica   Fold or ridge

Plicae semilunares   Folds (semicircular) into lumen of the large intestine

Plicae conniventes   Circular (complete circles) folds in the lumen of the small intestine; A.K.A. valvulae conniventes

Pneumaturia   Passage of urine containing air

Pneumothorax   Collapse of lung with **air** in pleural space

Pseudocyst   Dilated cavity resembling a true cyst, but **not** lined with epithelium

Pus   Liquid product of inflammation, consisting of dying leukocytes and other fluids from the inflammatory response

Rubor   Redness, classic sign of inflammation

Steatorrhea   Fatty stools due to decreased fat absorption (e.g., decrease in lipase secondary to pancreatitis)

Stenosis   Abnormal narrowing of a passage or opening

Sterile field   Area covered by sterile drapes or prepped in sterile fashion using antiseptics (e.g., Betadine)

Succus   Fluid derived from living tissue (e.g., succus entericus is fluid from the bowel lumen)

Tenesmus   Urge to defecate with ineffectual (and often painful) straining

Thoracotomy   Surgical opening of the chest cavity

Transect   To divide transversely (to cut in half)

Trendelenburg   Patient posture with pelvis higher than the head, inclined about 45°

Urgency   Sudden strong urge to urinate; often seen with a UTI

Wet to dry dressing Damp gauze dressing placed on wound and removed after the dressing dries to the wound; this provides microdebridement

SURGERY SIGNS AND TRIADS YOU SHOULD KNOW _____

Battle's sign

Ecchymoses over the mastoid process in patients with basilar skull fractures

Beck's triad

Seen in patients with cardiac tamponade:
1. JVD
2. Decreased or muffled heart sounds
3. Decreased blood pressure

Bergman's triad

Seen with fat emboli syndrome:
1. Mental status changes
2. Petechiae (often in the axilla/thorax)
3. Dyspnea

Blumer's shelf

Metastatic disease to the rectouterine (pouch of Douglas) or rectovesical pouch creating a "shelf" that is palpable on rectal exam

Bouchardt's triad

Seen with gastric volvulus:
1. Emesis
2. Epigastric pain
3. Inability to pass NG tube

Carcinoid triad

Seen with carcinoid syndrome:
1. Flushing
2. Diarrhea
3. R-sided heart failure

Charcot's triad

Seen with cholangitis:
1. Fever (chills)
2. Jaundice
3. RUQ pain

Courvoisier's law

An enlarged nontender gallbladder seen with obstruction of the common bile duct, most commonly seen with pancreatic CA. *Note:* not seen with acute cholecystitis as the gallbladder is scarred secondary to chronic cholelithiasis.

Cullen's sign

Bluish discoloration of the periumbilical area due to retroperitoneal hemorrhage tracking around to the anterior abdominal wall through fascial planes (i.e., in acute hemorrhagic pancreatitis)

Cushing's triad

Signs of increased intracranial pressure:
1. Hypertension
2. Bradycardia
3. Irregular respirations

Dance's sign

Empty RLQ in children with ileocecal intussusception

Fothergill's sign

Used to differentiate an intra-abdominal mass from one in the abdominal wall; if mass is felt while there is tension on the musculature, then it is in the wall (i.e., sitting halfway upright)

Grey Turner's sign

Ecchymosis or discoloration of the flank in patients with retroperitoneal hemorrhage (due to dissecting blood from the retroperitoneum)

Hamman's sign/crunch

Crunching sound on auscultation of the heart due to emphysematous mediastinum, seen with Boerrhaave's syndrome, pneumomediastinum, etc.

Homans' sign

Calf pain on forced dorsiflexion of the foot in patients with DVT

Howship-Romberg sign

Pain along the inner aspect of the thigh; seen with an obturator hernia due to nerve compression

Kehr's sign

Severe left shoulder pain often with LUQ pain in patients with splenic rupture (due to referred pain from diaphragmatic irritation)

Krukenburg tumor

Metastatic tumor to the ovary (classically from gastric CA)

Kelly's sign

Visible peristalsis of the ureter in response to squeezing or retraction; used to identify the ureter during surgery

Laplace's law

Wall tension = pressure × radius (thus, the colon perforates preferentially at the cecum, due to the increased radius and resultant increased wall tension)

Larrey's point

Subxiphoid

McBurney's point

$\frac{1}{3}$ the distance from the anterior iliac spine to the umbilicus on a line connecting the two

McBurney's sign

Tenderness at McBurney's point in patients with appendicitis

Meckel's diverticulum rule of 2's

2% of the population have a Meckel's diverticulum, 2% of those are symptomatic, and they occur approx. within 2 feet from the ileocecal valve

Mittelschmerz

Lower quadrant pain due to ovulation

Murphy's sign

Pain in the RUQ during inspiration, while palpating under the R costal margin. The patient cannot continue to inspire deeply, as it brings an inflamed gallbladder under pressure (seen in acute cholecystitis)

Obturator sign

Pain upon internal rotation of the leg with the hip and knee flexed, seen in patients with appendicitis/pelvic abscess

Psoas sign

Pain elicited by extending the hip with the knee in full extension, seen with appendicitis and psoas inflammation

Pheochromocytoma triad

1. Headache
2. Palpitations
3. Episodic diaphoresis

Raccoon eyes

Bilateral black eyes due to basilar skull fracture

Reynold's pentad

1. Fever
2. Jaundice
3. RUQ pain
4. Mental status changes
5. Shock/sepsis

Thus, Charcot's triad plus #4 & #5; seen in patients with suppurative cholangitis

Rovsing's sign

Palpation of the LLQ results in pain in the RLQ, seen in appendicitis, and helps differentiate abdominal source of pain from thoracic

Saint's triad	1. Cholelithiasis 2. Hiatal hernia 3. Diverticular disease
Sister Mary Joseph's sign (A.K.A. Sister Jeane Marie's sign or Sister Mary Joseph's node)	Metastatic tumor to umbilical lymph node(s)
Virchow's node	Metastatic tumor to left supraclavicular node (classically gastric CA)
Virchow's triad	Risk factors for thrombosis: 1. Stasis 2. Abnormal endothelium 3. Hypercoagulability
Westermark's sign	Decreased pulmonary vascular markings on CXR in a patient with pulmonary embolus
Whipple's triad	Evidence for insulinoma: 1. Hypoglycemia (< 50) 2. CNS and vasomotor Sx, i.e., syncope, diaphoresis, etc. 3. Relief of Sx's with administration of glucose

2
Common Operations

Billroth I   Antrectomy with gastroduodenostomy

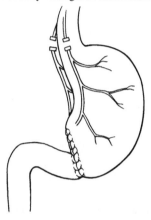

Billroth II   Antrectomy with gastrojejunostomy

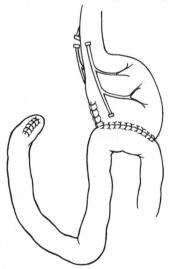

Roux-en-Y limb   Jejunojejunostomy forming a Y-shaped
figure of small bowel; the free end can then

be anastomosed to a second hollow structure (e.g., gastrojejunostomy)

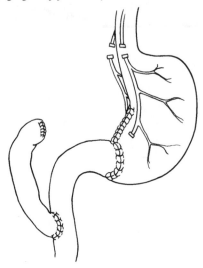

CEA	Carotid endarterectomy; removing the atherosclerotic plaque from a carotid artery
Bassini herniorrhaphy	Repair of inguinal hernia by approximating transversus abdominis aponeurosis and the conjoint tendon to the reflection of **Poupart's** (A.K.A. inguinal) ligament
McVay herniorrhaphy	Repair of inguinal hernia by approximating the transversus abdominis aponeurosis and the conjoint tendon to **Cooper's** ligament (basically the superior pubic bone periosteum)
Lichtenstein herniorrhaphy	"Tension-free" inguinal hernia repair utilizing **synthetic** graft material
Shouldice herniorrhaphy	Repair of inguinal hernia by **imbrication** of the transversalis fascia, transversus abdominis aponeurosis and the conjoint tendon and approximation of the transversus abdominis aponeurosis and the conjoint tendon to the inguinal ligament
APR	**A**bdomino**p**erineal **r**esection; removal of the rectum and sigmoid colon through abdominal and perineal incisions; patient is left with a colostomy
Anterior resection	Resection of the rectum through an anterior abdominal incision
Enterolysis	Lysis of peritoneal adhesions

Appendectomy   Removal of the appendix

Lap appy   Laparoscopic removal of the appendix

Cholecystectomy   Removal of the gallbladder

Lap chole   Laparoscopic removal of the gallbladder

Nissen   Nissen fundoplication; 360° wrap of the
                               stomach by the fundus of the stomach
                               around the distal esophagus to prevent reflux

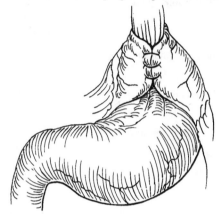

Modified radical mastectomy   Removal of the breast, nipple, and axillary
                                  lymph nodes (no muscle is removed)

Lumpectomy and radiation   Removal of breast mass and axillary lymph
                                  nodes; spares normal surrounding breast
                                  tissue; patient then undergoes postoperative
                                  radiation treatments

I and D   Incision and drainage; incision with drainage
                                  of pus—the wound is then packed open

PEG   Percutaneous endoscopic gastrostomy;
                                  endoscope is placed in stomach, stomach is
                                  inflated with air, needle is passed into
                                  stomach percutaneously, string is passed
                                  through abd wall, gastrostomy is then placed
                                  basically by using Seldinger technique

Exploratory laparotomy   Laparotomy to explore the peritoneal cavity
                                  looking for the cause of pain/peritoneal
                                  signs/obstruction/etc.

TURP   Transurethral resection of the prostate;
                                  removal of obstructing prostatic tissue via
                                  scope in the urethral lumen

Fem pop

Femoropopliteal artery bypass; femoral artery to popliteal artery bypass utilizing synthetic graft or saphenous vein; used to bypass blockage in the femoral artery

CABG

Coronary artery bypass grafting; via saphenous vein graft or internal mammary artery bypass grafts to coronary arteries from aorta = cardiac revascularization

Hartmann's pouch

Oversewing of a rectal stump (or distal colon stump) after resection of a colonic segment; patient is left with a proximal colostomy

Ileo-anal pull through

Anastomosis of ileum to anus after total colectomy

Hemicolectomy

Removal of a colonic segment, a partial colectomy

Truncal vagotomy

Transection of the vagus nerve trunks; must provide drainage procedure to stomach since after truncal vagotomy the pylorus does not relax (e.g., gastrojejunostomy or pyloroplasty)

Antrectomy

Removal of stomach antrum

Whipple procedure

Pancreaticoduodenectomy:

1. Cholecystectomy
2. Truncal vagotomy
3. Antrectomy
4. Pancreaticoduodenectomy = removal of the head of the pancreas and duodenum
5. Choledochojejunostomy (anastomosis of common bile duct to jejunum)
6. Pancreaticojejunostomy (anastomosis of distal pancreas remnant to the jejunum)
7. Gastrojejunostomy (anastomosis of stomach to jejunum)

3
Wounds, Drains, and Tubes

DEFINE _____

Primary wound closure? Immediate **suture wound closure**

Delayed primary closure? Suture closure of wound usually 3–5 days after incision (usually after wet to dry wound debridement)

Secondary wound closure? Wound closure over time **without sutures;** heals by contraction and epithelialization (leaves a large scar)

How long until a sutured wound epithelializes? ≈48 hours

What will inhibit wound healing? Malnutrition, anemia, hypoxia, steroids, cancer, radiation

What will reverse the deleterious effects of steroids on wound healing? Vitamin A

What is Dakin solution? Dilute sodium hypochlorite (A.K.A. **bleach**); use in contaminated (''soupy'') wounds

What is the purpose of drains?
1. Drainage of fluids
2. Apposition of tissues to remove a potential space by suction

What is a JP drain? **Jackson-Pratt drain;** a closed drainage system attached to a suction bulb (''grenade''); always remember to detach suction before pulling!

What is a Penrose drain? An open drainage system; basically, a thin rubber hose; associated with increased infection rates

DEFINE _____

G-Tube? **Gastrostomy tube;** for drainage or feeding

D-tube? **Duodenostomy tube;** for drainage, usually after duodenal trauma (rare)

23

J-tube?	**Jejunostomy tube;** for feeding, may be a small needle catheter (remember to flush after use or it will clog) or a large red rubber catheter
Cholecystostomy tube?	Tube placed surgically or percutaneously with ultrasound guidance to drain the gallbladder in patients with cholecystitis usually unable to withstand traditional surgery and in patients with acalculous cholecystitis
T-tube?	A tube placed in the common bile duct with an ascending and descending limb that forms a ''T''; drains percutaneously; usually placed after common bile duct exploration
When can one remove a T-tube?	Usually after 3 weeks; may remove if bilirubin level does not increase and there are no signs/Sx of cholangitis after clamping the T-tube
Why doesn't the bile duct leak bile after removal of a T-tube?	A fibrous tract forms around the T-tube prior to removal; the fibrous tract then scleroses down after removal of the T-tube, resulting in a patent and closed bile duct

DEFINE

Chest tube?	**Thoracostomy tube;** tube to drain the pleural cavity; attached to suction to appose the parietal and visceral pleura; used to drain blood/pus/fluid/chyle/air
Cecostomy tube?	Tube placed into cecum after colonic distention to decompress the colon; used basically in poor operative candidates after failed attempts of colonoscopic decompression

4
Surgical Anatomy Pearls

What is the drainage of the left testicular vein?　　Left renal vein

What is the drainage of the right testicular vein?　　IVC

What is the blood supply to the head of the pancreas?　　Branches of the gastroduodenal artery, and SMA (superior mesenteric artery): pancreaticoduodenal arteries

What is Gerota's fascia?　　Fascia surrounding the kidney; it often tamponades bleeding seen with blunt trauma to the kidney

What are the prominent collateral circulations seen in portal HTN?　　Esophageal varices, hemorrhoids (inferior hemorrhoidal v. to the internal iliac v.), patent umbilical vein (caput medusa), and retroperitoneal v. via lumbar tributaries

What parts of the GI tract are retroperitoneal?　　Most of the duodenum, the ascending colon, the descending colon, and the pancreas

What is the gubernaculum?　　Embryologic structure that adheres the testes to the scrotal sac; used to help manipulate the testes during indirect hernia repair

What artery bleeds in bleeding duodenal ulcers?　　Gastroduodenal artery

Name of lymph nodes between pectoralis minor and major muscles?　　Rotter's lymph nodes

Is the left vagus nerve anterior or posterior?　　Anterior; remember the esophagus rotates during development

What is Morrison's pouch?　　The hepatorenal recess; the most posterior cavity in the peritoneal cavity

DEFINE _____

Foregut?	Mouth to ampulla of Vater
Midgut?	Ampulla of Vater to distal $\frac{1}{3}$ of transverse colon
Hindgut?	Distal $\frac{1}{3}$ of transverse colon to the rectum
Where are the blood vessels on a rib?	The vein, artery, and nerve (''VAN'') are underneath the rib

5
Fluids and Electrolytes

Body fluid composition?	Fluids = 60% total body weight
	  40% ICF (intracellular)
	  20% ECF (extracellular)
	    15% Interstitial
	    5% Plasma

Average percentage body weight that is blood in the adult?	≈7%
Liters of blood in 70-kilogram man?	$0.07 \times 70 = 5$ liters
Fluid requirements every 24 hours?	Water = 30–35 ml/kg Sodium and potassium = 1 mEq/kg (Total = 60–80 mEq/24 hours) Chloride = 1.5 mEq/kg
Normal daily water losses?	1200–1500 ml urine (25–30 ml/kg) 200–400 ml sweat 500–700 ml respiratory losses 100–200 ml feces
Normal daily electrolyte losses?	Sodium and potassium = 100 mEq Chloride = 150 mEq (40 mEq/liter sodium and chloride lost as sweat)
Response to hypovolemia?	Sodium retention via renin→aldosterone, water retention via ADH, vasoconstriction via angiotensin II and sympathetics

THIRD SPACING

What is it?	Fluid accumulation in the interstitium of tissues as in edema; e.g., loss of fluid into the interstitium and lumen of a paralytic bowel following surgery (think of the intravascular and intracellular spaces as the first two spaces) *Note:* third-spaced fluid tends to mobilize back into the intravascular space around the

27

3rd post-op day; beware of overhydration once the fluid begins to return to the intravascular space

Signs?

Hypotension and dehydration

Rx?

IV hydration with isotonic fluids

Response to hypervolemia?

Decreased aldosterone secretion leading to decreased tubular reabsorption of Na and water excretion, ↓ angiotensin II, ↓ sympathetics

Surgical causes of metabolic acidosis?

Diarrhea, ileus, fistula, high-output ileostomy, renal tubular acidosis, carbonic anhydrase inhibitors (due to loss of bicarb); lactic acidosis, ketoacidosis, dehydration, renal failure, TPN

Surgical causes of metabolic alkalosis?

Vomiting, NG suction, diuretics, alkali ingestion, mineralocorticoid excess

Surgical causes of respiratory acidosis?

Hypoventilation (CNS depression), drugs (morphine), pneumothorax, pleural effusion, parenchymal lung disease, acute airway obstruction

Surgical causes of respiratory alkalosis?

Hyperventilation (anxiety, pain, fever, wrong ventilator settings)

What is paradoxic alkalotic aciduria?

Seen with hypokalemic, hypovolemic alkalosis (e.g., gastric fluid loss) as H^+ is lost in the urine in exchange for Na^+ in an attempt to restore volume; H^+ is exchanged preferentially instead of K^+, due to the low concentration of K^+

Changes in physical exam with volume derangements?

Weight changes, skin turgor, JVD, mucosal membranes

Changes in vital signs with hypovolemia?

Tachycardia, tachypnea, initial rise in diastolic blood pressure due to clamping down (peripheral vasoconstriction) with subsequent decrease in both systolic and diastolic bp.

What are the insensible fluid losses?

Feces: 100–200 ml/24 hr
Breathing: 500–700 ml/24 hr
Note: this increases with fever and tachypnea
Skin: approx. 300 ml/24 hr and increased with fever; thus, insensible fluid loss is not directly measured

What are the quantities of daily secretions?	Bile: approx. 1000 ml/24 hr Gastric: approx. 2000 ml/24 hr Pancreatic: approx. 600 ml/24 hr Small intestine: approx. 3000 ml/day Saliva: approx. 1500 ml/24 hr *Note:* almost all secretions are reabsorbed
Principles of fluid and electrolyte replacement?	1. Replace deficits 2. Fulfill daily maintenance requirements 3. Replace ongoing losses
Common IV replacement fluids	All values are per liter
What is in normal saline? (NS)	154 mEq of Cl^- 154 mEq of Na^+
What is in $\frac{1}{2}$ NS?	77 mEq of Cl^- 77 mEq of Na^+
What is in $\frac{1}{4}$ NS?	39 mEq of Cl^- 39 mEq of Na^+
What is in lactated Ringer's (LR)?	130 mEq Na^+ 110 mEq Cl^- 28 mEq lactate 4 mEq K^+ 3 mEq Ca^+
D5W	5% dextrose (50 grams) in H_2O
What accounts for tonicity?	Mostly electrolytes; thus NS and LR are both isotonic while $\frac{1}{2}$ NS is hypotonic
What happens to lactate in LR in the body?	The lactate is converted into bicarbonate; thus, LR cannot be used as a maintenance fluid because patients would get alkalotic

CALCULATION OF MAINTENANCE FLUIDS

100/50/20 Rule?	Maintenance IV fluids for 24-hour period 100 ml/kg for first 10 kg 50 ml/kg for next 10 kg 20 ml/kg for every kg > 20 kg (divide by 24 for hourly rate)
4/2/1 Rule?	Maintenance IV fluids—hourly rate 4 ml/kg for first 10 kg 2 ml/kg for next 10 kg 1 ml/kg for every kg >20 kg

Maintenance for a 70-kg man?	Using 100/50/20:
	    100×10 kg = 1000
	    50×10 kg = 500
	    20×50 kg = 1000
	    total = 2500
	    divided by 24 hr:
	    104 ml/hr maintenance rate
	Using 4/2/1:
	    4×10 kg = 40
	    2×10 kg = 20
	    1×50 kg = 50
	    total = 110 ml/hr maintenance rate

Common adult maintenance fluid?	D5 ½ NS with 20 mEq KCl/liter
Common pediatric maintenance fluid?	D5 ¼ NS with 20 mEq KCl/liter (use ¼ NS because of decreased ability of children to concentrate urine)
Why add sugar to maintenance fluid?	To inhibit muscle breakdown
Best way to assess fluid status?	Urine output (unless the patient has cardiac or renal dysfunction, in which case central venous pressure or wedge pressure is best)
Minimal UO for adult on maintenance IV?	≥30 ml/hr urine output (UO)
Minimal UO for adult trauma patient?	≥50 ml/hr
Number of ml in 12 oz?	356 ml
Number of ml in 1 oz?	30 ml
Number of ml in 1 tsp?	5 ml

ELECTROLYTE IMBALANCES

Common cause of electrolyte abnormalities?	Lab error!

HYPERKALEMIA _____

Surgical causes?	Iatrogenic overdose, blood transfusion, renal failure, diuretics, acidosis, tissue destruction (injury/hemolysis), insulin deficiency

Signs/Sx?	Decreased DTRs (deep tendon reflex) or arreflexia, weakness, parasthesia, paralysis, respiratory failure
EKG findings?	**Peaked T waves,** depressed ST segment, prolonged PR, wide QRS, bradycardia, ventricular fib → asystole
Critical value?	$K^+ > 6.5$: EKG monitoring required $K^+ > 7.0$: Rx is urgent
Urgent Rx?	1. Calcium gluconate IV (cardioprotective) 2. Sodium bicarbonate IV (alkalosis drives K^+ intracellularly) 3. Glucose and insulin 4. Kayexalate and **Lasix** (if not hypovolemic) 5. Dialysis: peritoneal vs. hemodialysis
Nonacute Rx?	Lasix and/or Kayexalate

HYPOKALEMIA

Surgical causes?	Diuretics, certain antibiotics, steroids, alkalosis, diarrhea, intestinal fistulae, NG aspiration, vomiting, insulin, insufficient supplementation
Signs/Sx?	Weakness, tetany, N/V, **ileus,** parasthesia
EKG findings?	PAC, PVC, flattening of T waves, U waves, ST segment depression
Rapid Rx?	KCl IV
Slow Rx?	KCl PO

HYPERNATREMIA

Surgical causes?	Inadequate hydration, diabetes insipidus, diuresis, vomiting, diarrhea, diaphoresis, tachypnea
Signs/Sx?	Seizures, confusion, stupor, pulmonary or peripheral edema, tremors, respiratory paralysis
Rx:	
1. Hypovolemic?	Rehydrate with NS (then D5W)

2. **Euvolemic?**   D5W IV slowly (prevent cerebral edema)

3. **Hypervolemic?**   (Rare) Lasix followed by D5W

HYPONATREMIA _____

Surgical causes?

1. **Hypovolemic?**   Diuretic excess, hypoaldosteronism,
                                            vomiting, NG suction, burns, pancreatitis,
                                            diaphoresis

2. **Euvolemic?**   SIADH, CNS abnormalities, drugs

3. **Hypervolemic?**   Renal failure, CHF, liver failure (cirrhosis),
                                            iatrogenic fluid overload (dilutional)

Signs/Sx?   Seizures, coma, N/V, ileus, lethargy,
                                            confusion, weakness

Rx:

1. **Hypovolemic?**   NS IV, correct underlying cause

2. **Euvolemic?**   SIADH: Lasix and NS acutely, fluid restrict

3. **Hypervolemic?**   Dilutional: fluid restriction and diuretics

''PSEUDOHYPONATREMIA'' _____

What is it?   Spurious lab value of hyponatremia due to
                                            hyperglycemia and/or hyperproteinemia

HYPERCALCEMIA _____

Causes?   Causes (DDx) of hypercalcemia:
                                            ''C.H.I.M.P.A.N.Z.E.E.S.''
                                              Calcium supplementation IV
                                              Hyperparathyroidism (1°/2°/3°)
                                                Hyperthyroidism
                                              Immobility/**I**atrogenic (thiazide diuretics)
                                              Mets/**M**ilk alkali syndrome
                                              Paget's disease (bone)
                                              Addison's disease/**A**cromegaly
                                              Neoplasm (colon, lung, breast, prostate,
                                                multiple myeloma)
                                              Zollinger-Ellison syndrome (as part of
                                                MEN I)
                                              Excessive vitamin D
                                              Excessive vitamin A
                                              Sarcoid

Signs/Sx?	Hyperparathyroidism: ''Stones, bones, abdominal groans, and psychiatric overtones''
ECG findings?	Short QT interval, prolonged PR interval
Acute Rx?	Volume expansion with NS, diuresis with Lasix (not thiazides), steroids, calcitonin, phosphate, dialysis
Chronic Rx?	Restrict calcium intake, steroids, phosphate

HYPOCALCEMIA _____

Surgical causes?	Short bowel syndrome, intestinal bypass, vitamin D deficiency, acute pancreatitis, osteoblastic metastasis, aminoglycosides, diuretics, renal failure, medullary CA-thyroid (ectopic secretion of calcitonin)
Chvostek's sign?	Facial muscle spasm with tapping of facial n.
Trousseau's sign?	Carpal spasm after occluding blood flow in forearm with BP cuff.
Signs/Sx?	Chvostek's and Trousseau's sign, parasthesia (early) and increased DTRs (late), confusion, abdominal cramps, laryngospasm, stridor, seizures, tetany, psych. abnormalities (paranoia, depression, hallucinations)
EKG findings?	Prolonged QT interval
Acute Rx?	Calcium gluconate IV
Chronic Rx?	Calcium PO, vitamin D

HYPERMAGNESEMIA _____

Surgical cause?	TPN
Signs/Sx?	Respiratory failure, CNS depression, decreased DTRs (Remember, on ob?)
Treatment?	Calcium gluconate IV, insulin + glucose, dialysis (similar to Rx for hyperkalemia)

HYPOMAGNESEMIA _____

Surgical cause?	TPN
Signs/Sx?	Increased DTRs, tetany, asterixis, tremor, Chvostek's sign, ventricular ectopy, vertigo, tachycardia

Acute Rx?	$MgSO_4$ IV
Chronic Rx?	Magnesium oxide PO (side effect: diarrhea)

HYPERGLYCEMIA

Surgical causes?	Diabetes (poor control), infection, stress, TPN, drugs, lab error (drawing over IV site)
Signs/Sx?	Polyuria, hypovolemia, confusion/coma, polydipsia, ileus, DKA (Kussmaul breathing), abdominal pain, hyporeflexia
Treatment?	IVF, insulin, monitor glucose and electrolytes

HYPOGLYCEMIA

Surgical causes?	Excess insulin, decreased caloric intake, insulinoma, drugs, liver failure, adrenal insufficiency
Signs/Sx?	Sympathetic response (diaphoresis, tachycardia, palpitations), confusion, coma, headache, diplopia, neurologic deficits, seizures
Treatment?	Glucose IV or PO
How does one correct for the Ca^{2+} level in hypoalbuminemia?	(4 minus the measured albumin level) $\times\ 0.8$ and add this to the measured Ca^{2+} level to get the corrected level

MISCELLANEOUS ELECTROLYTE QUESTIONS

This EKG pattern is consistent with what electrolyte abnormality?	*HYPERKALEMIA:* Peaked T-waves

If hyperkalemia is left untreated what can it lead to?	Ventricular tachycardia/fibrillation → death

6
Blood and Blood Products

What is . . .

Whole blood?	One unit = 450 ml (±50 ml); deficient in platelets and clotting factors V, VIII, and XI; rarely used
Packed red blood cells (PRBC)?	One unit = 300 ml (±50 ml); no platelets or clotting factors; can be mixed with NS to infuse faster
Platelets (plts)?	Replaces platelets; one (random donor) unit ≈ 50 ml; usually infuse 6–8 units or one single donor unit (250–300 ml)
Fresh frozen plasma (FFP)?	Replaces clotting factors; no RBCs/WBCs/plts
Cryoprecipitate (cryo)?	Replaces fibrinogen and some clotting factors
Which electrolyte is most likely to fall with the infusion of stored blood? Why?	Ionized calcium; the citrate preservative used for the storage of blood binds serum calcium
What changes occur in the storage of whole blood? (7)	$\downarrow Ca^{2+}$, $\uparrow K^+$, $\downarrow$ 2,3-DPG, $\uparrow H^+$ ($\downarrow$ pH), $\downarrow$ clotting factors (V, VII, & XI), $\downarrow$ PMNs
Rough formula to convert Hgb to Hct?	Hbg × 3 ≈ Hct
One unit PRBC $\uparrow$ Hct by how much?	≈3–4%

7
Common Surgical Medications

ANTIBIOTICS

What do first, second, and third generation cephalosporin refer to in regard to spectrum?

Gram-negative activity, with third-generation having the most

DEFINE

Cefazolin

1st generation; surgical prophylaxis for **skin flora**

Cefoxitin

2nd generation; used for mixed aerobic/anaerobic infections; *Bacteroides fragilis* coverage; has **anaerobic** coverage!

Ceftazidime

3rd generation, with best activity against *Pseudomonas*

Clindamycin

Strong activity against Gram-negative **anaerobes** such as *Bacteroides fragilis*

Gentamicin

Aminoglycoside used for **Gram-negative** coverage; nephrotoxic, ototoxic; follow blood peak/trough levels

Imipenem

Last resort against serious, multiresistant organisms; (**covers about everything**) usually combined with cilastin, which inhibits the renal excretion of imipenem

Metronidazole

Serious **anaerobic** infections (e.g., diverticulitis) also used to Rx amebiasis; patient must abstain from alcohol use during therapy

Mezlocillin

An anti-pseudomonal penicillin with good **Enterobacteriaceae** activity; commonly used for cholangitis because it covers the common biliary tract organisms

Nafcillin

Antistaphylococcal penicillin commonly used for cellulitis

Vancomycin	Treat methicillin-resistant *Staphylococcus aureus* (MRSA). PO Vanc: treat *C. difficile* pseudomembranous colitis (poorly absorbed from gut); follow peak/trough levels with IV Rx; ototoxicity/nephrotoxicity, ''red man syndrome'' = flushing—correct by slow infusion
Meperidine	Injectable narcotic; used commonly with acute pancreatitis/biliary pathology as morphine may cause sphincter of Oddi spasm/constriction

STEROIDS

Side effects (>10)?	Adrenal suppression, immunosuppression, weight gain with central obesity, cushingoid facies, acne, hirsutism, purple striae, hyperglycemia, sodium retention/ hypokalemia, hypertension, osteopenia, myopathy, ischemic bone necrosis (avascular necrosis of the hip), gastrointestinal perforations
Uses?	Immunosuppression—transplant, autoimmune diseases; hormone replacement—Addison's disease; spinal cord trauma, etc. **Never acutely stop steroids—always taper.**
Who needs ''stress dose'' steroids before surgery?	Every patient who is on steroids, suspected hypoadrenal, or before adrenalectomy

HEPARIN

Action?	Binds with and **activates antithrombin III;** follow **pTT** level and maintain about 1½ to 2 times normal
Uses?	Pulmonary embolism, prophylax/treat deep vein thrombosis, stroke, atrial fibrillation—prophylax embolism, acute occlusion of an artery; low molecular wgt sub Q: prophylaxis for DVT
Side effects?	Bleeding complications; can cause thrombocytopenia!
Reverse with?	**Protamine** IV (1 : 100, 1 mg of protamine to every 100 units of heparin)

Half life?	About 90 minutes
Stop how long before surgery?	4–6 hours preop

COUMADIN

Action?	**Inhibits vitamin K–dependent clotting factors II, VII, IX, X,** (i.e., 2, 7, 9, 10) produced in the liver; follow PT levels, maintain at 1.5–2.0 times normal
Uses?	Long-term anticoagulation (PO)
Caution?	Bleeding complications
Half life?	**48 hours!** thus if you change a dose one day, don't expect a change in the PT the next day! wait 2 days!
Reverses with?	**Cessation,** vitamin K, fresh-frozen plasma (in emergencies)
Stop how long before surgery?	Stop 3–5 days preop and start on IV heparin, then stop the heparin 4–6 hours preop; can then restart heparin postop and start back on coumadin in a few days

DEFINE _____

Sucralfate	Treats peptic ulcers by forming an acid-resistant barrier; binds to ulcer craters; needs acid to activate—thus do not use with H2 blocker!
Cimetidine	H_2 blocker: ulcers/gastritis
Ranitidine	H_2 blocker: ulcers/gastritis
Omeprazole	Gastric acid secretion inhibitor; works by inhibiting the K^+/H^+-ATPase (*Note:* causes carcinoid tumors in rats!)
Promethazine	Acute antinausea med—use postop
Metoclopramide	Increase gastric emptying with increase in LES pressure; dopamine antagonist; use in diabetic gastroparesis and to help move feeding tubes past the pylorus
Albumin	Expands plasma volume, 5% albumin; 25% albumin—draws extravascular fluid into intravascular space indicated in severe hypoalbuminemia

8
Complichions

RESPIRATORY COMPLICATIONS

ATELECTASIS

What is it?	Collapse of the alveoli
Etiology?	Inadequate alveolar expansion; i.e., poor ventilation of lungs during surgery, inability to fully inspire secondary to pain, excessive sputum retarding air flow
Signs?	Fever, decreased breath sounds with rales present, tachypnea, tachycardia, and increased density on CXR
Risks?	COPD, smoking, abdominal or thoracic surgery
Claim to fame?	**Most common cause of postop fever during POD 1–2
Prophylaxis?	Cessation of smoking at least two days prior to OR, incentive spirometry
Rx?	Postop deep breathing, coughing, postural drainage, suctioning, and incentive spirometry

POSTOP RESPIRATORY FAILURE

What is it?	RR >25 pH <7.20 pCO_2 >50 pO_2 <60 *Note:* these values are approximations
DDx?	Hypovolemia, pulmonary embolism, impaired respiratory drive with administration of O_2 to a patient with chronic CO_2 retention (i.e., COPD), atelectasis, pneumonia, increased intraabdominal pressure, pneumothorax, chylothorax, hemothorax, narcotic overdose (give Narcan)
Rx?	O_2 and intubate/ventilate if necessary

Possible causes of postop pleural effusion?	Diaphragmatic inflammation with possible subphrenic abscess formation, fluid overload

PULMONARY EMBOLISM

What is it?	Blood clot from the venous system (usually lower extremity or pelvic veins is site of origin) that embolizes to the pulmonary arterial system
Risk factors?	Postoperative, immobility, CHF, obesity, use of oral contraceptives, neoplastic disease, advanced age, polycythemia, MI
Signs/Sx?	SOB, tachypnea, hypotension, CP, occasionally fever, tender LE, loud pulmonic component of S2
Labs?	ABG: decreased pO_2 and pCO_2 (from hyperventilation)
Dx tests?	V-Q scan (ventilation—perfusion scan), CXR (which may show Westermark's sign—wedge-shaped area of decreased pulmonary vasculature and infarction); pulmonary A-gram is the gold standard; TEE is newest diagnostic test
Rx?	Anticoagulation, Greenfield filter if anticoagulation is contraindicated or if patient has further PE on adequate anticoagulation (consider thrombolysis or embolectomy in severe cases)

ASPIRATION PNEUMONIA

What is it?	Pneumonia following aspiration of vomitus
Risks?	Intubation/extubation, impaired consciousness, (i.e., drug or ETOH overdose), dysphagia (esophageal disease), nonfunctioning NGT, Trendelenburg position
Signs/Sx?	Respiratory failure, CP, increased sputum production, fever, cough, mental status changes, tachycardia, cyanosis
CXR?	Early—fluffy infiltrate Late—pneumonia, ARDS
Commonly involved lobe?	Supine—RUL Sitting/semirecumbant—RLL

Common organisms?	Community acquired: Gram +/mixed Hospital/ICU: Gram − rods
Dx?	CXR, sputum Gram stain, sputum culture, bronchoalveolar lavage
Rx?	Bronchoscopy, abxs if pneumonia develops, intubation if respiratory failure, ventilate with PEEP if ARDS develops
What is Mendelson's syndrome?	Chemical pneumonitis secondary to aspiration of the stomach contents (i.e., gastric acid), abx not necessary unless bacterial infection arises

GASTROINTESTINAL COMPLICATIONS

NG tube complications	1. Aspiration—pneumonia/atelectasis
	2. Sinusitis
	3. Minor UGI bleeding
	    —epistaxisis
	    —pharyngeal irritation

GASTRIC DILATATION

Risk factors?	Abdominal surgery, gastric outlet obstruction, splenectomy
Signs/Sx?	Abdominal distension, hiccups, electrolyte abnormalities, and nausea
Rx?	NG tube decompression

POSTOPERATIVE PANCREATITIS

What is it?	Pancreatitis due to manipulation of the pancreas during surgery or low blood flow during the procedure (i.e., cardiopulmonary bypass)
Rx?	Same as other causes of pancreatitis (i.e., NPO, ±NG tube, fluid resuscitation, etc.)

SHORT BOWEL SYNDROME

What is it?	Malabsorption and diarrhea resulting from extensive bowel resection (approx. ≤100 cm of small bowel remaining)
Initial Rx?	TPN early, followed by many small meals chronically

Postop SBO

Causes?	Adynamic ileus, incarcerated hernia intussusception, adhesions (most of which resolve spontaneously)
Signs of resolving ileus?	Flatus PR, stool, abdominal cramping, increasing appetite, bowel sounds
Order of recovery of bowel function after abdominal operation?	1st—small intestine 2nd—stomach 3rd—colon

Causes of Postop Jaundice?

Prehepatic?	Hemolysis (prosthetic valve), resolving hematoma, transfusion reaction, post-cardiopulmonary bypass, blood transfusions (decreased RBC compliance leading to cell rupture)
Hepatic?	*Drugs,* hypotension, hypoxia, sepsis, hepatitis, ''sympathetic'' hepatic inflammation from adjacent RLL infarction of the lung or pneumonia, preexisting cirrhosis, R-sided heart failure, hepatic abscess, pylephlebitis (thrombosis of portal vein), Gilbert's, Crigler-Nager, and Dubin-Johnson syndromes, fatty infiltrate from TPN
Posthepatic?	Obstruction (stone), cholangitis, cholecystitis, biliary duct injury, pancreatitis, sclerosing cholangitis; tumors: cholangiocarcinoma, pancreatic CA, gallbladder CA, metastases
What blood tests would support the assumption that hemolysis was causing jaundice in a patient?	**Decreased:** Haptoglobin, Hct **Increased:** LDH, reticulocytes also fragmented RBCs on a peripheral smear

Blind Loop Syndrome

What is it?	Bacterial overgrowth in the small intestine. The organisms that tend to overgrow are not the normal flora of the small bowel (such as Gram-positive, aerobic organisms resembling oropharyngeal flora). Rather, they are more representative of colonic flora (such as Gram-negative bacteria like *Escherichia coli.*) In fact, there is often overgrowth of

strictly anaerobic bacteria like *Clostridium* and *Bacteroides* species.

Causes?

Anything that disrupts the normal flow of intestinal contents (i.e., causes stasis), stricture of the intestine, Crohn's disease, postvagotomy syndromes, scleroderma, small bowel diverticula, decreased gastric acid secretion, incompetent ileocecal valve

Signs/Sx?

Diarrhea, steatorrhea, malnutrition, abdominal pain, hypocalcemia, megaloblastic anemia (due to B_{12} deficiency)

Pathogenesis of B12 deficiency?

Two hypotheses:
1. Bacterial utilization of B_{12}
2. Bacterial toxins inhibit the absorption of B_{12} across the small bowel mucosa

Diagnostic tests?

Schilling test: demonstrating an intrinsic factor–resistant B_{12} malabsorption
Hydrogen breath test: lactose is swallowed and expiration of H_2 is monitored. With bacterial overgrowth there is increased H_2 production earlier than is normal

Treatment?

Surgical correction of the underlying disorder causing the stasis if feasible, otherwise antibiotics to inhibit bacterial overgrowth

Other causes of B_{12} deficiency?

Gastrectomy (decreased secretion of intrinsic factor) and excision of the terminal ileum (site of B_{12} absorption)

AFFERENT LOOP SYNDROME

What is it?

Partial or total obstruction/kink of the afferent limb following a Billroth II, with accumulation of bile and pancreatic secretions in the afferent limb

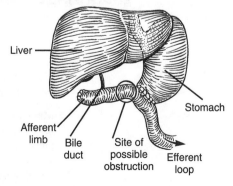

Liver

Stomach

Afferent limb   Bile duct   Site of possible obstruction   Efferent loop

Signs/Sx?	Postprandial RUQ pain and bilious vomiting, anemia, steatorrhea; pain often resolves suddenly after decompression of afferent limb
When does it present?	Approx. 66% present in the first week postop; otherwise it can occur anytime
Dx?	UGI in which the afferent loop will not fill with contrast due to the obstruction
Rx?	Balloon dilatation, surgical reanastomosis (e.g., Roux-en-Y)

DUMPING SYNDROME

What is it?	Delivery of *hyperosmotic* chyme to the small intestine causing massive fluid shifts into the bowel (normally the stomach will decrease the osmolality of the chyme prior to its emptying)
Associated with what conditions?	Any procedure that bypasses the pylorus or compromises its function (i.e., gastroenterostomies or pyloroplasty); thus, "dumping" of chyme into small intestine
Signs/Sx?	Postprandial diaphoresis, tachycardia, abdominal pain/distention, emesis, increased flatus, dizziness, weakness
Dx?	History, hyperosmolar glucose load will elicit similar Sx
Rx?	Small, multiple, low fat/carbohydrate meals that are high in protein content; also **avoidance of liquids** with meals to slow gastric emptying—surgery is a last resort

ENDOCRINE COMPLICATIONS

SIADH

What is it?	Syndrome of inappropriate antidiuretic hormone secretion, which results in excessive fluid retention (think of *i*nappropriate *i*ncrease)
Causes?	**Mainly lung/CNS:** CNS trauma, oat cell lung CA, pancreatic CA, duodenal CA, pneumonia/lung abscess, increased PEEP, CVA, general anesthesia, idiopathic postoperative, morphine

Labs?	Low sodium, low chloride, low serum osmolality, and increased urine osmolality
Rx?	Treat the primary cause and **restrict** fluid intake

DIABETES INSIPIDUS

What is it?	Decreased release of ADH resulting in massive I's and O's (think of *D*iabetes = *D*ecreased ADH)
Risks?	Head trauma
Rx?	IV vasopressin to replace the deficiency and massive quantities of IV fluids

ADDISONIAN CRISIS

What is it	Acute adrenal insufficiency in the face of a *stressor* (i.e., surgery, trauma, or infection); the normal response of increased glucocorticoid release is impaired
Signs/Sx?	Nausea, vomiting, diarrhea, ***abdominal pain,*** ± fever, progressive lethargy, ***hypotension,*** **eventual hypovolemic shock**
Labs?	Decreased sodium, increased K^+ (secondary to decreased aldosterone)
Rx?	IVFs (D5 NS), *Cortisol IV*

CARDIOVASCULAR COMPLICATIONS

Arterial line complications?	Infection, thrombosis which can lead to finger necrosis, death/hemorrhage due to catheter disconnection. **Remember to perform and document the *Allen test* before inserting an arterial line or obtaining a blood gas sample
What is an Allen test?	To test adequate collateral blood flow to the hand via the ulnar artery: patient clenches fist; you then occlude both radial and ulnar arteries; patient then opens the blanched hand. Release the ulnar artery. If the palm has an immediate strong blush, the ulnar artery should be adequate collateral flow if the radial a. thromboses

Dyspnea following central line placement

Common causes?	Pneumothorax, pericardial tamponade, carotid puncture (which can cause a hematoma that compresses the trachea), air embolism
DDx of postop chest pain?	MI, atelectasis, pneumonia, pleurisy, esophageal reflux, pulmonary embolism, musculoskeletal pain, subphrenic abscess, aortic dissection, pneumo/chylo/hemothorax
DDx of postop atrial fibrillation?	**Fluid overload, PE, MI, pain** (excess catecholamines), atelectasis, pneumonia, digoxin toxicity, hypoxemia, thyrotoxicosis (remember George Bush), hypercapnia, idiopathic

MYOCARDIAL INFARCTION

Risk of reinfarction following noncardiac surgery:

Time of Previous MI	Risk of Infarction
<3 Months ago	30% (50% mortality)
4–6 Months ago	15% (33% mortality)
>6 Months ago	7% (33% mortality) *Note:* risk decreases by about 50% every 3 months

When do postop MIs occur?	⅔ occur on postop days 2–5 (are often silent and present with **dyspnea**)

RENAL/COAGULATION/FAT EMBOLI COMPLICATIONS

FAT EMBOLI SYNDROME

What is it?	Embolization of fat particles
Risks?	Fractures of the long bones, trauma
Signs?	**Bergman's triad** (mental status changes, petechiae, and dyspnea); CXR picture similar to ARDS as fat particles cause a pneumonitis

Complications?   Respiratory failure, DIC

Rx?   Ventilatory support with PEEP as necessary, steroids (controversial), diuretics, and Rx of DIC if it develops

POSTOPERATIVE RENAL FAILURE _____

What is it?   Urine output <25 ml/hr (30 ml/hr is minimum adult output), increased creatinine, increased BUN

DDx?   Prerenal: inadequate fluids, hypotension
Renal: acute tubular necrosis, nephrotoxic dyes or drugs
Postrenal: Foley catheter obstruction/stone

Indications for dialysis?   Fluid overload, refractory hyperkalemia, BUN >130, acidosis

DISSEMINATED INTRAVASCULAR COAGULATION _____

What is it?   Activation of the coagulation cascade by a substance leading to thrombosis and consumption of clotting factors (esp. factors V and VIII) and platelets, which results in bleeding and fibrinolysis

Causes?   Tissue necrosis, septic shock, massive large vessel coagulation, shock, allergic reactions, blood transfusion reaction, cardiopulmonary bypass, cancer, obstetric complications, snakebites

Signs/Sx?   Diffuse bleeding from incision sites, venipuncture sites, catheter sites, or mucous membranes; also acrocyanosis or other signs of thrombosis

Lab Dx?   Increased fibrin degradation products, elevated PT/PTT, decreased platelets, decreased fibrinogen (level correlates well with bleeding), presence of schistocytes (fragmented RBCs) increased D-dimer.

Rx?   **Removal of the cause,** otherwise supportive; IVFs, O_2, platelets, FFP, cryoprecipitate (fibrin) as needed
Use of heparin is controversial, but may be indicated in a picture that is predominantly thrombotic

9
Common Causes of Ward Emergencies

Causes of hypotension?

Hypovolemia (iatrogenic, hemorrhage), myocardial infarction, cardiac arrhythmia, hypoxia, false reading (wrong cuff/arterial line twist or clot, etc.), pulmonary embolus, cardiac tamponade (on thoracic service), morphine (histamine release)

Hypertension: common causes in postop setting?

Pain (from catecholamine release), anxiety, hypercapnia, hypoxia (which may also cause hypotension) idiopathic/preexisting

Causes of hypoxia?

Atelectasis, pneumonia, mucous plug, pneumothorax, pulmonary embolus, myocardial infarction/arrhythmia, venous blood in ABG syringe, SAT% machine malfunction/probe malposition, iatrogenic (wrong ventilator settings), severe anemia/ hypovolemia, low cardiac output

Mental status change?

Hypoxia until ruled out, hypotension (cardiogenic shock, etc.), hypovolemia, iatrogenic (narcotics/benzo), drug reaction, alcohol withdrawal, drug withdrawal, seizure, ICU psychosis in ICU, CVA, sepsis, metabolic derangements, intracranial bleeding, urinary retention in the elderly

Signs of ETOH withdrawal?

Confusion, tachycardia/autonomic instability, seizure, hallucinations

10
Surgical Nutrition

What is the motto of surgical nutrition?	If the gut works—use it.

Normal daily dietary requirements for adults:
  Protein?
  Calories?
	
	1 gm/kg/day
	35 kcal/kg/day

By how much is basal energy expenditure (BEE) ↑ or ↓ in the following:
  Severe head injury?
  Severe burns?
	
	Increased $\approx 1.7 \times$
	Increased $\approx 2-3 \times$

What are the calorie contents and metabolic by-products of the following:
  Fat?
  Protein?
  Carbohydrate?
	
	9 kcal/gm; $CO_2 + H_2O$
	4 kcal/gm; ammonia
	4 kcal/gm; $CO_2 + H_2O$

Formula for the conversion of nitrogen requirement/loss to protein requirement/loss?	Nitrogen $\times$ 6.25 = protein
What is RQ?	Respiratory quotient: the ratio of CO_2 produced to O_2 consumed
What dietary change can be made to decrease CO_2 production in a patient in whom CO_2 retention is a concern?	Decrease carbohydrate calories and increase calories from fat
Lab tests to monitor nutritional status? (6)	Evidence of poor nutrition: ↓ PREALBUMIN (T$\frac{1}{2} \approx$ 2–3 days). ↓ Transferrin (T$\frac{1}{2} \approx$ 8–9 days). ↓ Albumin (T$\frac{1}{2} \approx$ 14–20 days). Total lymphocyte count < 1800. Anergy ↓ Retinol binding protein (T$\frac{1}{2} \approx$ 12 hours)
Where is iron absorbed?	Duodenum (some in proximal jejunum)

Where is vitamin B$_{12}$ absorbed?	Terminal ileum
Surgical causes of vitamin B$_{12}$ deficiency? (3)	Gastrectomy, excision of terminal ileum, blind loop syndrome
Where are bile salts absorbed?	Distal 200 cm of ileum
Where are fat-soluble vitamins absorbed?	Terminal ileum
Which vitamins are fat soluble?	K, A, D, E ("KADE")
What are the signs of:	
Vitamin A deficiency?	Poor wound healing
Vitamin B$_{12}$/folate deficiency?	Megaloblastic anemia
Biotin deficiency?	Rash, neuromuscular sx, ECG changes
Vitamin C deficiency?	Poor wound healing, bleeding gums
Vitamin K deficiency?	↓ in the vitamin K–dependent clotting factors (II, VII, IX, and X); bleeding
Chromium deficiency?	Diabetic state, especially in patients with AODM
Selenium deficiency?	Anergy
Zinc deficiency?	Poor wound healing, alopecia, dermatitis, taste d/o
Fatty acid deficiency?	Dry, flaky skin; alopecia
What vitamin increases the PO absorption of iron?	PO vitamin C (ascorbic acid)
What vitamin lessens the deleterious effects of steroids on wound healing?	Vitamin A
Common indications for total parenteral nutrition (TPN)?	NPO > 7 days Enterocutaneous fistulas Short bowel syndrome Pancreatitis
Complications of TPN?	Line infection, fatty infiltration of the liver, electrolyte/glucose problems, pneumothorax during placement of central line, loss of gut barrier
Advantages of enteral feeding?	Keeps gut barrier healthy, thought to lessen translocation of bacteria, no complications of line placement, fewer electrolyte/glucose problems
What is the major nutrient of the gut?	Glutamine

11
Shock

Definition?	Inadequate tissue perfusion
Classification of types?	1. Hypovolemic 2. Septic 3. Cardiogenic 4. Neurogenic 5. Anaphylactic
Signs?	Skin: pale, diaphoretic, cool Hypotension, ↓ mental status Tachycardia Poor capillary refill Poor urine output, tachypnea
Best indicators of tissue perfusion?	Blood pressure, urine output, mental status, capillary refill

TYPES OF SHOCK

HYPOVOLEMIC SHOCK _____

Definition?	Decreased intravascular volume
Common Causes?	Hemorrhage Burns Bowel obstruction Crush injury Pancreatitis
Signs?	Early: Orthostatic hypotension Mild tachycardia, anxiety Diaphoresis Vasoconstriction (decreased pulse pressure with increased diastolic pressure) Late: Changed mental status Decreased blood pressure Marked tachycardia
Classification of hypovolemic shock?	**Mild:** (20% or less blood volume loss), decreased perfusion to nonvital tissues, manifested by pale, cool skin, anxiety

51

Moderate: (20–40% blood volume loss) decreased perfusion to vital tissues (liver, kidneys, intestine), manifested by olig-/anuria and decreased BP, agitation
Severe: (40% or greater blood volume loss), decreased perfusion to brain and heart, manifested by mental status changes and cardiac irregularities

Treatment?

IVF and blood via one or more IVs; the most effective initial fluid in restoring intravascular volume is isotonic crystalloid (normal saline/lactated Ringer's).
Of course, as the resuscitation is in progress the underlying cause of hypovolemia should be identified and treated.

Evaluation of effectiveness of treatment?

Most useful indicator: urine output
Also useful:
central venous pressure, blood pressure, heart rate, Hct, ABG, mental status, capillary refill, wedge pressure

Failure of resuscitation?

Usually due to persistent massive hemorrhage, requiring emergent surgical procedure

SEPTIC SHOCK

Definition?

Decreased vascular resistance, decreased intravascular volume usually due to septicemia causing increased capillary permeability and microvascular pooling and most likely cardiac dysfunction

Specific etiology?

Most Common: Gram neg septicemia
Less Common: Gram pos septicemia

What increases the susceptibility to septic shock?

Any mechanism that increases the susceptibility to infection, i.e., trauma, immunosuppression, corticosteroids, hematologic disease, diabetes

What is a major risk in septic shock?

Disseminated intravascular coagulation, **death**

Signs/Sx?

Initial: vasodilation resulting in warm skin and full pulses, normal urine output
Delayed: vasoconstriction and poor urine output, mental status changes, hypotension

Associated findings?

Fever, hyperventilation

Lab tests?

Early: 1. Hyperglycemia/glycosuria
      2. Respiratory alkalosis
      3. Hemoconcentration
      4. Leukopenia
Late: Leukocytosis
Important to identify organism to direct treatment

Treatment?

1. IVFs → blood cultures
2. Antibiotic therapy
   a. vs. identified organism
   b. empirical if org. unknown
3. Drainage: Surgical drainage of an abscess or focus of infection, because antibiotics will not suffice.
4. Pressors PRN

CARDIOGENIC SHOCK

Definition?

Cardiac insufficiency, usually left ventricular failure, resulting in inadequate tissue perfusion

Signs/Sx?

Note: Clinical findings are often minimal, yet anticipate those of congestive heart failure and MI
On exam:
1. Dyspnea
2. Rales
3. Pulsus alternans (increased pulse with greater filling following a weak pulse)
4. Loud pulmonic component of S2
5. Gallop rhythm

Signs on chest x-ray?

Pulmonary venous congestion

Treatment?

Based on diagnosis/mechanism:
1. Congestive heart failure: diuretics and vasodilators
2. Left ventricular failure (myocardial infarction)
   a) low LV filling pressure, nl cardiac output, low blood pressure, treat with IVFs
   b) increased LV filling pressure, nl cardiac output, nl blood pressure, treat by diuresis
   c) nl LV filling pressure, low cardiac output, increased blood pressure, treat with vasodilation to reduce resistance to LV ejection

NEUROGENIC SHOCK

Definition?	Inadequate tissue perfusion due to loss of sympathetic vasoconstrictive reflexes

Common causes?	1. Spinal trauma
	   a. Complete transection
	   b. Partial cord injury with spinal shock
	2. Spinal anesthesia
	3. Vasodilator drugs
	4. Fright/anxiety

Signs/Sx?	Pallor, weakness, lightheadedness, transient **hypotension and bradycardia** (prior to compensation by increased cardiac activity)
Associated findings?	Neurologic deficits suggesting cord injury, rapid stabilization with resuscitation
Treatment?	*IV fluids*
What percentage of hypotensive patients with spinal neurologic deficits have hypotension of purely neurogenic origin?	about ⅔
What is spinal shock?	Complete flaccid paralysis immediately following spinal cord injury; this may or may not be associated with circulatory shock
What is the lowest reflex available to the examiner?	Bulbocavernous reflex: checking for contraction of the anal sphincter upon compression of the glans penis or clitoris
What is the lowest level voluntary muscle?	External anal sphincter

ANAPHYLACTIC SHOCK

Definition?	Inadequate tissue perfusion due to increased vascular permeability, vasodilation, smooth muscle constriction as a result of exposure to an allergen in a previously sensitized individual
Most important part of evaluation? (Always)	History
What are the most common causes of anaphylactic death in the U.S.?	1. Medications 2. Hymenoptera venom (bee sting) 3. Food/blood transfusions

Associated findings?

Skin: Urticaria and angioedema
Airway: Laryngeal edema resulting in airway obstruction
Lungs: Smooth muscle constriction resulting in respiratory distress with wheezing
Intest: Mucosal edema causing nausea, vomiting, diarrhea, and crampy abd pain

Treatment?

1. Establish airway
2. Epinephrine
3. Benadryl, if epinephrine is inadequate
4. Steroids
5. Aminophylline

12
Surgical Infection

Elements common to surgical infections?	1. An infectious agent 2. Susceptible host 3. Closed unperfused space (ischemic)
What is a superinfection?	New infection arising while patient is receiving antibiotics (abx) for the original infection at a different site; due to resistant bacteria
What is a UTI?	Urinary tract infection
Dx?	Urine dipstick, culture, urine microscopy for WBC
# of CFU for Dx?	On urine culture, classically 100,000 or 10^5 colony forming units
Common organisms?	*E. coli, Klebsiella, Proteus*
Rx?	Abx
Rx bladder candidiasis?	Amphotericin bladder washings
Signs of a cental line infection?	**Unexplained hyperglycemia,** fever, mental status change, hypotension, tachycardia → SHOCK
Rx?	Remove line/abx
Wound infection	
Signs/Sx?	**Pain** at incision site, erythema, drainage
Rx?	Remove skin sutures/staples, digital examination to rule out fascial dehiscence, pack wound open
What is bacterial translocation?	Bacteria gain access to lymphatics and blood stream from colon via compromised mucosal barrier

Classification of Operative Wounds

What is a "clean" wound?	Elective, nontraumatic wound without acute inflammation; usually closed primarily without the use of drains

What is the infection rate of a clean wound?	<1.5%
What is a clean contaminated wound?	Operation of the GI or respiratory tract without unusual contamination, or entry into the biliary or urinary tract
Without infection present, what is the infection rate of a clean-contaminated wound?	<3%
What is a contaminated wound?	Acute inflammation present, a traumatic wound, GI tract spillage, or a major break in sterile technique
What is the infection rate of a contaminated wound?	Approx. 5%
What is a dirty wound?	Pus present, perforated viscus, or dirty traumatic wound
What is the infection rate of a dirty wound?	Approx. ⅓!
Complications of wound infections?	Fistulas, sinus tracts, sepsis, abscess, suppressed wound healing, superinfections (i.e., a new infection that develops during antibiotic Rx for the original infection)
Factors influencing the development of infections?	—Presence of a foreign body, i.e., suture, drains, grafts, etc. —Decreased blood flow (poor delivery of PMNs and antibiotics) —Strangulation of tissues with excessively tight sutures —Presence of necrotic tissue or excessive local tissue destruction (e.g., too much Bovie) —Long operations (>2 hr) —Hematomas or seromas —Presence of dead space that prevents the delivery of phagocytic cells to bacterial foci —Poor approximation of tissues
Patient factors	—Uremia —Hypovolemic shock —Vascular occlusive states —Old age

—Immunosuppressed states: immunosuppressant Rx, chemotherapy, systemic malignancy, trauma or burn injury, diabetes mellitus, obesity, malnutrition, AIDS

What is an abscess?

—Localized collection of pus and fibrin surrounded by an area of inflammation (i.e., hyperemia and marked leukocyte infiltration)
—CT may aid in the diagnosis
—Abscess always requires drainage, which can be either surgical or percutaneous if the anatomic location of the abscess is accessible (except hepatic amebiasis!)

Labs?

Leukocytosis or leukopenia (as an abscess may act as a WBC sink), blood cultures, imaging studies (i.e., CT to locate an abscess)

Rx?

1. Incision and drainage—an abscess must be drained (I&D). *Note:* fluctuation is a sign of a subcutaneous abscess. Most abdominal abscesses are drained percutaneously.
2. Antibiotics

PSEUDOMEMBRANOUS COLITIS

What is it?

Antibiotic-induced colonic overgrowth of *C. difficile,* secondary to loss of competitive nonpathogenic bacteria that comprise the normal colonic flora
Note: it can be caused by any ABX, but especially penicillins and cephalosporins

Signs/Sx?

Diarrhea, ± fever, ± increased WBC, ± abdominal cramps, ABD distention

Cause of the diarrhea?

Exotoxin released by *C. difficile*

Dx?

**Assay stool for exotoxin titer; fecal leukocytes may or may not be present; on colonoscopy there is an exudate that looks like a membrane and thus ''pseudomembraneous''

Rx?

PO vancomycin (97% sensitive) or PO Flagyl (93% sensitive); stop causative agent
Never give antiperistaltics. Cholestyramine will bind the exotoxin and may help alleviate the diarrhea.

Prophylactic Antibiotics _____

Risk/benefits	One must weigh the possible benefit against possible adverse effects (i.e., allergic rxn's, superinfections, e.g., *C. difficile* for example)
Indications for prophylaxis? (IV abx)	1. Accidental wounds with heavy contamination and tissue damage 2. Accidental wounds requiring surgical therapy that has had to be delayed 3. Injuries where adequate debridement cannot be performed 4. Known gross bacterial contamination in any wound 5. Penetrating injuries of hollow intraabdominal organs 6. Lg bowel resections and anastomosis (PO neomycin plus erythromycin on the day prior to surgery, and cefoxitin preop) 7. Some clean-contaminated procedures (i.e., common bile duct exploration) 8. Patient with preexisting valvular heart disease 9. Cardiovascular surgery with the use of a prosthesis/vascular procedures 10. Patients with open fractures (in ER) 11. Traumatic wounds occuring >8 hr prior to medical attention
What must a prophylactic antibiotic cover for procedures on the large bowel/ABD trauma?	Must cover anaerobes!
Commonly used antibiotics with anaerobic coverage?	Cefoxitin, clindamycin, metronidazole,
Timing of prophylactic antibx?	Antibiotic must be in adequate levels in the blood stream PRIOR TO SURGICAL INCISION!

PAROTITIS _____

What is it?	Inflammation of the parotid gland
Common bacteria?	Staphylococci
Risks?	>65 years old, malnutrition, poor oral hygiene, presence of NG tube; NPO, dehydration

Time of occurrence?	Usually 2 weeks postop
Signs?	Hot, red, tender parotid gland, and increased WBC
Rx?	Antibiotics, operative drainage prn
Bacteria make up what percentage of the dry weight of feces?	About ⅓
What is the antibiotic of choice for *Actinomyces*?	Penicillin G (exquisitely sensitive)
What is a furuncle?	A staphylococcal abscess that forms in a hair follicle (*F*ollicle = *F*uruncle)
What is a carbuncle?	A subcutaneous staphylococcal abscess (usually an extension of a furuncle), most commonly seen in diabetics (i.e., R/O diabetes)
What is suppurative hidradenitis?	Infection of an apocrine sweat glands (therefore seen in the axilla, perineum, and inguinal distributions)
What microscopic finding is associated with *Actinomyces*?	Sulfur granules
What organism causes tetanus?	*Clostridium tetani*
What are the signs of tetanus?	Lockjaw, muscle spasm, laryngospasm, convulsions, and respiratory failure
Tetanus prophylaxis in tetanus-prone injury	
Previous immunization × 3?	Tetanus toxoid
No previous immunization?	Tetanus immunoglobulin IM and tetanus toxoid IM (at different sites!)
What is Fitz-Hugh-Curtis syndrome?	RUQ pain due to gonococcal perihepatitis in women

13

Fever

Define postoperative fever	Temperature >38.5°C
What are the classic W's of postoperative fever? (5)	Wind—atelectasis POD #1–2 Wound—wound infection POD 5–7 Water—UTI Walking—DVT thrombitis Wonder drugs—drug fever
Causes of fever during op or immediately postop?	Malignant hyperthermia—familial reaction to halothane or succinylcholine Transfusion reaction, drug hypersensitivity, atelectasis, aspiration pneumonia, and endocrine (addisonian crisis, thyroid storm, pheochromocytoma)
Fever before 24-hr postop?	Atelectasis, streptococcal or clostridial wound infections (rare) *Note:* S.T.A.T. = strep, thyroid, addisonian, transfusion
Most common cause of fever POD 1–2?	**Atelectasis!**
Causes of fever 3–5 days postop?	—UTI—especially after instrumentation/ Foley —Pneumonia —IV complications; rate of infection is proportional to the duration of IV site (thrombophlebitis/central line sepsis) —Wound complications: leaking anastamosis, hematoma, etc.
Causes of fever 6–10 days PO?	Wound infection, pneumonia, abscess, infected hematoma, *C. difficile* colitis
Deep venous thrombosis (DVT), abscess, drug fever	Pulmonary embolism, abscess, parotitis
The following can cause fever at any time:	—Thrombophlebitis —Pulmonary embolus/DVT —Drug hypersensitivity —Transfusion reaction —UTI —Central line sepsis

14
Surgical Prophylaxis

Protection from postoperative GI bleeding?

H2 blockers (e.g., ranitidine or cimetidine), Carafate (binds ulcer craters), or antacids

Protection from postoperative atelectasis/pneumonia?

Incentive spirometry, coughing, **stop smoking** (even if for 48 hr!)

Protection from postoperative deep venous thrombosis?

Subcutaneous low-dose heparin and/or sequential compression device (SCD) for lower extremities, support hose

Protection from wound infection?

Shower night before surgery with chlorhexidine scrub. **Never use razor** for hair removal (electric shavers only). Adequate skin prep in *OR*. Do not close the skin in a contaminated case. Preoperative antibiotic in bloodstream before incision. Leave wound open if contaminated case.

Protection from fungal infection while on IV antibiotics?

PO nystatin

Protection from infection after colon surgery?

Lower bacterial count in colon by catharsis and PO antibiotics preoperatively

15
Surgical Radiology

Percentage of kidney stones that are radiopaque?	≈90%
Percentage of all gallstones that are radiopaque?	≈10%
Percentage of radiopaque fecaliths present in appendicitis?	≈5%
Signs of abdominal pathology on abdominal x-ray (AXR)?	Loss of fat stripe, loss of psoas shadow, sentinel loops, cutoff sign, air-fluid levels, free air
Radiographic signs of appendicitis?	Fecalith, sentinal loops, scoliosis away from the right due to pain, mass effect (abscess), loss of psoas shadow, loss of preperitoneal fat stripe, and very rarely a small amount of free air if perforated
Best x-ray for diagnosing an AAA?	Cross-table lateral—reveals AAA in >⅔ by eggshell calcifications
What does KUB stand for?	Kidneys, ureters, and bladder: commonly used term for a plain film x-ray of the abdomen
CXR findings that may provide evidence of traumatic aortic injury?	**Widened mediastinum****! Apical pleural capping Central sign of congestion Pleural fluid Broken ribs (esp. 1st or 2nd) Loss of aortic knob Inferior displacement of left main bronchus; NG tube displaced to the right, tracheal deviation, large hemothorax
What is the parrot's beak or bird's beak sign? (2)	Evidence of sigmoid volvulus on barium enema; evidence of achalasia on barium swallow

Differential diagnosis of retroperitoneal calcification? (6)

Pancreatitis, AAA, generalized aortic calcification, kidney stone, renal cell carcinoma, renal artery aneurysm (phleboliths if seen in pelvis)

Differential diagnosis and best position for the detection of free peritoneal air?

Seen in any intraabdominal viscus perforation, s/p laparotomy, s/p needle bx, s/p paracentesis, or rarely from the female reproductive tract (such as after water-skiing); **upright CXR** or left lateral decubitus, since this prevents confusion with gastric air bubble; with free air BOTH sides of the bowel wall can be seen; can detect as little as 1 cc of air

What is the significance of an air-fluid level?

Seen in obstruction or ileus on an upright x-ray; intraluminal bowel diameter increases, allowing for separation of fluid and gas

What is meant by a "cutoff sign"?

Seen in obstruction, bowel distention, and air-fluid level that is "cut off" from normal bowel

What are "sentinal loops"?

Distention and/or air-fluid levels near a site of abdominal inflammation (e.g., seen in the RLQ with appendicitis)

What is loss of the psoas shadow?

Loss of the clearly defined borders of the psoas muscle on AXR; loss signifies inflammation or ascites

What is loss of the peritoneal fat stripe?

(A.K.A. preperitoneal fat stripe) loss of the lateral peritoneal/preperitoneal fat interface; implies inflammation

How can one tell if bowel on AXR is small or large bowel?

By the intraluminal folds; the small bowel plicae circulares are complete, while the plica semilunares of the large bowel are only partially around the inner circumference of the lumen

16
Anesthesia

Local anesthesia	Anesthesia of a small confined area of the body (i.e., lidocaine for an elbow laceration)
Epidural anesthesia	Anesthetic drugs/narcotics infused into epidural space
Spinal anesthesia	Anesthetic agents injected into the thecal sac
Regional anesthesia	Blocking sensory afferent nerve fibers from a region of the body (i.e., radial nerve block)
General anesthesia	Unconsciousness/amnesia (inhalational anesthetics)

NAME EXAMPLES OF

Local anesthetic	Lidocaine, buvipicaine
Regional anesthetic	Lidocaine, buvipicaine
General anesthesia	Halothane, isoflurane, enflurane, nitrous oxide
Dissociative agent	Ketamine (children/burn patients)
What is cricoid pressure?	Manual pressure on cricoid cartilage occluding esophagus and thus decreasing chance of aspiration of gastric contents
What is rapid-sequence anesthesia induction?	1. Short-acting IV barbiturate (thiopental most common) 2. Muscle relaxant 3. Cricoid pressure 4. Intubation 5. Inhalation anesthetic (rapid: boom, boom, boom → to lower risk of aspiration during intubation)
Contraindications of the depolarizing agent succinylcholine?	Burn patients, trauma, neuromuscular diseases/paraplegia

Why is succinylcholine contraindicated in these patients?	Depolarization in these patients can result in life-threatening **hyperkalemia**
Side effect of the nonpolarizing neuromuscular blocker pancuronium?	Tachycardia
Why doesn't lidocaine work in an abscess?	Lidocaine does not work in an acidic environment
Why does lidocaine burn on injection and what can be done to decrease the burning sensation?	Lidocaine is acidic, which causes the burning; add sodium bicarb to decrease the burning sensation
Why does some lidocaine come with epinephrine?	Epinephrine is meant to vasoconstrict the small vessels and thus decrease bleeding and decrease the washout of the lidocaine from the area, prolonging its effect
Where is lidocaine with epinephrine contraindicated?	Fingers, toes, penis, etc.; because of possibility of ischemic injury/necrosis due to vasoconstriction
Contraindications to nitrous oxide?	Nitrous oxide is poorly soluble in serum and thus expands into any air-filled body pockets; thus, try to avoid in cases with middle ear occlusions, **pneumothorax, small bowel obstruction,** etc.
What is the feared side effect of buvipicaine?	Cardiac arrhythmia after intravascular injection
Side effects of morphine?	Constipation, respiratory failure, hypotension (from histamine release), spasm of sphincter of Oddi (use Demerol in pancreatitis and biliary surgery), decreased cough reflex *Note:* life-threatening side effects can be reversed with **Naloxone**
Side effects of meperidine?	Similar to those of morphine, except causes less sphincteric spasm, but can cause seizures
Side effects of epidural analgesia?	**Orthostatic hypotension,** decreased motor function, urinary retention; advantage—analgesia without decreased cough reflex
Side effect of spinal anesthesia?	**Urinary retention** Hypotension (neurogenic shock)

Side effect of inhalational (volatile) anesthesia?	Halothane: HYPOTENSION (cardiac depression, decreased baroreceptor response to hypotension, and peripheral vasodilation), malignant hyperthermia

MALIGNANT HYPERTHERMIA

What is it?	Inherited predisposition to an anesthetic Rxn, causing uncoupling of the excitation-contraction system in skeletal muscle, which in turn causes *malignant* **hyperthermia;** hypermetabolism will result in death if untreated
Incidence?	Very rare
Causative agents?	General anesthesia, succinylcholine—*Note:* it is *not* associated with barbiturates, narcotics, or nitrous oxide
Signs/Sx?	**Increased body temp,** hypoxia, acidosis, tachycardia, leading to death if untreated
When does it occur?	Usually soon after the induction of the anesthetic
Rx?	*IV dantrolene,* body cooling, stop anesthesia

SECTION II
General Surgery

17
Acute Abdomen and Referred Pain

What are peritoneal signs?

Signs of peritoneal irritation including extreme tenderness, rebound tenderness (tenderness upon release of pressure after palpation), voluntary guarding (tightened abdominal muscles with palpation), pain with movement such as rocking the patient's pelvis or by striking heel of the patient, decreased or absent bowel sounds, and involuntary guarding/rigidity late

If a patient has peritoneal signs who must be called?

A **general surgeon!**

What Dx must be considered in every patient with an acute abdomen?

Appendicitis!

DDx BY QUADRANTS

RUQ

Cholecystitis, hepatitis, PUD, perforated ulcer, pancreatitis, liver tumors, gastritis, hepatic abscess, choledocholithiasis, cholangitis, pyelonephritis, nephrolithiasis, appendicitis ****(esp. during pregnancy)**; thoracic causes—pleurisy/pneumonia, PE, pericarditis, MI (esp. inferior MI)

LUQ

PUD, perforated ulcer, gastritis, splenic disease or rupture, abscess, reflux, dissecting aortic aneurysm, thoracic causes as above, pyelonephritis, nephrolithiasis, hiatal hernia (strangulated paraesophageal hernia), Boerhaave's syndrome, Mallory-Weiss tear

LLQ

Diverticulitis, sigmoid volvulus, perforated colon, colon CA, UTI, SBO, IBD, nephrolithiasis, pyelonephritis, fluid accumulation from aneurysm or perforation, referred hip pain; GYN causes—**ectopic pregnancy, PID, mittelschmerz, ovarian cyst, fibroid degeneration, endometriosis, GYN tumor, torsion of cyst or fallopian tube

RLQ	Same as LLQ, especially **appendicitis,** also mesenteric lymphadenitis, cecal diverticulitis, Meckel's diverticulum, intussusception
Causes of diffuse abdominal pain?	Uremia, porphyria, diffuse peritonitis, gastroenteritis, IBD, DKA, early appendicitis, SBO, sickle cell crisis, ischemic mesenteric disease, aortic aneurysm, lead poisoning, black widow spider bite, pancreatitis, perforated viscus
Causes of suprapubic pain?	Cystitis, colonic pain, GYN causes
Pain limited to specific dermatomes?	Early zoster before vesicles erupt
Pain in any quadrant?	Abscess or infection
What is referred pain?	Pain felt at a site distant from a disease process; due to the convergence of multiple pain afferents in the posterior horn of the spinal cord

CLASSIC LOCATIONS OF REFERRED PAIN? _____

Cholecystitis	Right subscapular pain (also epigastric)
Appendicitis	Early—periumbilical Rarely—testicular pain
Diaphragmatic irritation (from spleen, perforated ulcer, or abscess)	Shoulder pain (on the left a + Kehr's sign)
Pancreatitis/CA	Back pain
Rectal disease	Pain in small of back
Nephrolithiasis	Testicular pain/flank pain
What lab test should every woman with an acute abdomen of childbearing age receive?	β-HCG (human chorionic gonadotropin)

18
Hernias

What is a hernia?	The protrusion of an organ or tissue out of the body cavity in which it normally lies
Incidence?	5–10% lifetime incidence; 50% are indirect inguinal, 25% are direct inguinal hernias, and about 15% are femoral hernias
Precipitating factors?	Increased intraabdominal pressure: Straining at defecation or urination (rectal CA, colon CA, prostatic enlargement, constipation), obesity, pregnancy, ascites, valsavagenic (coughing) COPD; the presence of an abnormal congenital anatomical route (i.e. patent processus vaginalis)

DESCRIPTIVE TERMS

Reducible	The ability to return the displaced organ or tissue/hernia contents to its usual anatomic site
Incarcerated	Swollen or fixed within the hernia sac; may or may not cause intestinal obstruction (incarcerated = imprisoned) i.e., an irreducible hernia
Strangulated	Incarcerated hernia with resulting ischemia; will result in signs and Sx of ischemia and intestinal obstruction (i.e., pain and vomiting); think strangulated = choked.
Complete	Hernia sac and its contents protrude all the way through the defect
Incomplete	Defect present without sac or contents protruding completely through it

TYPES OF HERNIAS?

Sliding hernia	The hernia sac is partially formed by the wall of a viscus (i.e., bladder/cecum)
Littre's hernia	Hernia involving a Meckel's diverticulum

Spigelian hernia	Hernia through the linea semilunaris (or spigelian fascia); A.K.A. spontaneous lateral ventral hernia
Internal hernia	Hernia into or involving intraabdominal structure
Obturator hernia	Hernia through obturator canal (female > male)
Lumbar hernia	Petit's hernia or Grynnfeltt's hernia
Petit's hernia	Hernia through Petit's triangle (rare) A.K.A. inferior lumbar triangle (think, petit = small = inferior)
Grynnfeltt's hernia	Hernia through Grynfelt-Lesshaft triangle (superior lumbar triangle)
Pantaloon hernia	Hernia sac exists as both a direct and indirect hernia straddling the inferior epigastric vessels and protruding through the floor of the canal as well as the internal ring
Richter's hernia	Incarcerated or strangulated hernia involving only one wall of the bowel, which can spontaneously reduce, resulting in gangrenous bowel and perforation within the abdomen without signs of obstruction
Incisional hernia	Hernia through an incisional site; most common cause is a wound infection
Ventral hernia	Incisional hernia in the ventral abdominal wall; *Note:* obesity is associated with recurrence
Epigastric hernia	Hernia through the linea alba above the umbilicus
Umbilical hernia	Hernia through the umbilical ring, associated with ascites, pregnancy, and obesity
Intraparietal hernia	Hernia where abdominal contents migrate between the layers of the abdominal wall
Properitoneal hernia	Intraparietal hernia between the peritoneum and the transversalis fascia
Cooper's hernia	Hernia involving femoral canal and tracts into the scrotum or labia majus

Indirect inguinal	Inguinal hernia lateral to Hesselbach's triangle
Direct inguinal	Inguinal hernia within Hesselbach's triangle
Hiatal hernia	Hernia through the esophageal hiatus
What are the boundaries of Hesselbach's triangle?	1. **Inferior epigastric vessels** 2. **Inguinal ligament** (Poupart's) 3. **Lateral border of the rectus sheath**
What are the boundaries of Petit's triangle?	(A.K.A. inferior lumbar triangle) Posteriorly—**latissimus dorsi** Anteriorly—**external oblique** Inferiorly—**iliac crest** Floor consists of internal oblique and the transversus abdominis muscle
What are the boundaries of Grynnfeltt-Lesshaft's triangle?	(A.K.A. superior lumbar triangle) Superiorly—**12th rib** Anteriorly—**internal oblique** Floor—**quadratus lumborum**
What are the layers of the abdominal wall?	Skin Subcutaneous fat Scarpa's fascia Ext. oblique Internal oblique Transversus abdominus Transversalis fascia Preperitoneal fat Peritoneum *Note:* all three muscle layer aponeuroses form the anterior rectus sheath, with the posterior rectus sheath being deficient below the arcuate line

DIRECT INGUINAL HERNIA

What is it?	A hernia within the floor of Hesselbach's triangle, i.e., the hernia sac does not traverse the internal ring (think of directly through the abdominal wall)
Cause?	Acquired defect from mechanical breakdown over the years
Incidence?	Approximately 1% of all males, with frequency increasing with advanced age

What nerve runs with the spermatic cord in the inguinal canal?	Ilioinguinal nerve *(L2)*

INDIRECT INGUINAL HERNIA

What is it?	Hernia through the internal ring of the inguinal canal, traveling down toward the external ring; it may enter the scrotum upon exiting the external ring (i.e., if complete); think of the hernia sac traveling indirectly through the abdominal wall from the internal ring to the external ring
Cause?	Patent processus vaginalis (i.e., congenital)
Incidence?	Approx. 5% of all males—most common hernia in both males and females
Dx of inguinal hernia?	Relies mainly on history and PE with index finger invaginated into the external ring and palpation of hernia; examine patient standing up if Dx not obvious; *Note:* if swelling occurs below the inguinal ligament it is most likely a femoral hernia
DDx of inguinal hernia?	Inguinal adenitis, femoral adenitis, psoas abscess, ectopic testis, hydrocele of the cord, saphenous varix, lipoma
Risk of strangulation?	Higher with indirect than direct inguinal hernia, but highest in femoral hernias
Rx?	Emergent herniorrhaphy indicated if strangulation present or impending; otherwise, elective herniorraphy indicated to prevent chance of incarceration → strangulation.

FEMORAL HERNIA

What is it?	Hernia traveling beneath the inguinal ligament down the femoral canal medial to the femoral vessels
Associations?	Women, pregnancy, and exertion
Incidence?	Greater in females than males, but indirect inguinal still most common in females
Complications?	Approx. $\frac{1}{3}$ incarcerate (due to narrow, unforgiving neck)

What is the most common hernia in females?	Indirect inguinal hernia

ESOPHAGEAL HIATAL HERNIAS

Types?	1. Paraesophageal 2. Sliding

PARAESOPHAGEAL HIATAL HERNIA

What is it?	Herniation of stomach or part of it through the esophageal hiatus into the thorax without displacement of gastroesophageal junction; A.K.A. type II hiatal hernia
Incidence?	<5% of all hiatal hernias (rare)
Sx	Derived from mechanical obstruction—dysphagia, stasis gastric ulcer, and strangulation; many are asymptomatic and not associated with reflux because of relatively normal position of GE junction
Complications?	Hemorrhage, incarceration, obstruction, and strangulation
Rx?	Surgical because of frequency and severity of potential complications

SLIDING ESOPHAGEAL HIATAL HERNIA

What is it?	Both the stomach and the GE junction herniate into the thorax via the esophageal hiatus; A.K.A. type I hiatal hernia
Incidence?	>90% of all hiatal hernias
Sx?	Majority asymptomatic, but can cause REFLUX, dysphagia (from inflammatory edema), esophagitis, and pulmonary problems secondary to aspiration
	Reflux is due to the displacement of the GE junction into the thorax; this results in loss of the normal contribution from intraabdominal pressure to the competency of the LES as the intrathoracic pressure is 10–15 mm Hg lower
Dx?	UGI series, manometry, EGD with bx for esophagitis

Complications?	Reflux → esophagitis → Barrett's esophagus → cancer and stricture formation; aspiration pneumonia; it can also result in UGI bleeding from esophageal ulcerations
Rx?	85% of cases Rx'd medically with antacids, head elevation after meals, small meals, no food prior to sleeping; 15% of cases require surgery for persistent Sx despite adequate medical Rx; Nissen fundoplication involves wrapping the fundus around the LES and suturing it in place; this maintains the LES intraabdominally and helps buttress the sphincter

HERNIA REVIEW QUESTIONS

What is the most common hernia in females?	Indirect inguinal hernia
Perform elective TURP or elective herniorrhaphy first?	TURP first
Which type of esophageal hiatal hernia is associated with GE reflux?	Sliding esophageal hiatal hernia

19
Laparoscopy

What is laparoscopy?	Minimally invasive surgical technique utilizing gas to insufflate the peritoneum and instruments manipulated through ports introduced through small incisions
What gas is used?	CO_2
Which operations are done with the laparoscope?	Frequently: cholecystectomy, appendectomy, hernia repair, liver biopsy, many gyn operations including tubal ligation & laparoscopic assisted vaginal hysterectomy, many urologic procedures (including retroperitoneal lymphadenectomy) Not so frequently: bowel resection, colostomy, Nissen fundoplication, surgery for PUD, colectomy
Contraindications?	Absolute: hypovolemic shock, intestinal obstruction, large pelvic or abdominal mass, severe cardiac decompensation Relative: peritonitis, multiple previous surgical procedures, diaphragmatic hernia, COPD
Complications?	Pneumothorax, bleeding, perforating injuries, infection, intestinal injuries, solid organ injury, vascular injury
Advantages over laparotomy?	Shorter hospitalization, less pain & scar, lower cost, decreased ileus
Steps in laparoscopic cholecystectomy?	1. Dissection of peritoneum overlying cystic duct & artery 2. Clipping of cystic artery & cannulation of cystic duct 3. Intraoperative cholangiogram if necessary 4. Division of cystic duct between clips 5. Dissection of gallbladder from liver bed 6. Cauterization, irrigation, suction to get hemostasis of liver bed 7. Removal of gallbladder through umbilical trocar site

How to verify that the Verres needle is in the peritoneum?

Syringe of saline: saline should flow freely without pressure through the needle "Drop Test"

If Verres needle is not in peritoneal cavity what happens to the CO$_2$ flow/ pressure?

Flow decreases and pressure is way up

What is the Hasson technique?

No Verres needle—cut down and place trocar under **direct visualization**

20
Trauma

Trauma care in the United States follows what widely accepted protocol?	The ATLS (Advance Trauma Life Support) precepts of the American College of Surgeons
What are the three main elements of the ATLS protocol?	1. Primary survey/resuscitation 2. Secondary survey 3. Definitive care
What about the patient history?	Should be obtained while completing the primary survey; often the rescue squad, witnesses, and family members must be relied upon

PRIMARY SURVEY

What are five steps of the primary survey?	
A?	Airway
B?	Breathing
C?	Circulation
D?	Disability
E?	Exposure (You *must* know these!)
What principles are followed in completing the primary survey?	Life-threatening problems discovered during the primary survey are *always* addressed *before* proceeding to the next step.

Airway

What are the goals during assessment of the airway?	Securing the airway and protecting the spinal cord
In addition to the airway what *must* be considered during the airway step?	Spinal immobilization if there is any question of spinal injury
What comprises adequate spinal immobilization?	Use of a full backboard and rigid cervical collar

In an alert patient, what is the quickest test for an adequate airway?	Ask a question; if the patient can speak the airway is intact
What is the first maneuver used to establish an airway?	Chin lift and/or jaw thrust; if successful, often an oral or nasal airway can be used to temporarily maintain the airway
If these methods are unsuccessful what is the next maneuver used to establish an airway?	Endotracheal intubation, either nasal or oral
Contraindication to nasotracheal intubation?	**Maxillofacial fracture!**
If all other methods are unsuccessful what is the definitive airway?	Cricothyroidotomy, either by percutaneous placement of a needle through the cricothyroid membrane or by surgical placement of a tube through the cricothyroid membrane = "surgical airway"
What must always be kept in mind during difficult attempts at establishing an airway?	Spinal immobilization and adequate oxygenation; if at all possible, patients must be adequately ventilated with 100% oxygen using a bag and mask before any attempt at establishing an airway

BREATHING

What are the goals in assessing breathing?	Securing oxygenation and ventilation and treatment of life-threatening thoracic injuries
What comprises adequate assessment of breathing?	Inspection: for air movement, respiratory rate, cyanosis, tracheal shift, jugular venous distention, asymmetric chest expansion, use of accessory muscles of respiration, open chest wounds Auscultation: for upper airway sounds (stridor, wheezing, or gurgling), and for lower airway sounds present over both lung fields Percussion: hyperresonance or dullness over either lung field Palpation: presence of subcutaneous emphysema, flail segments
What are six life-threatening conditions that *must* be diagnosed and treated during the breathing step?	Airway obstruction, tension pneumothorax, open pneumothorax, flail chest, cardiac tamponade, massive hemothorax

How does one diagnose and treat tension pneumothorax?

Diagnosis: dyspnea, tachypnea, anxiety, pleuritic chest pain, unilateral decreased or absent breath sounds, tracheal shift away from the affected side, hyperresonance on the affected side; tension pneumothorax is a clinical Dx!
Treatment: **immediate** decompression by **needle thoracostomy** in the second intercostal space midclavicular line, followed by **tube thoracostomy** placed in the anterior/midaxillary line in the 4th intercostal space (level of the nipple in males)

How does one diagnose and treat open pneumothorax, also known as sucking chest wound?

Diagnosis: usually obvious, with air movement through a chest wall defect
Treatment in ER: intubation with positive-pressure ventilation, tube thoracostomy (chest tube), dressing

How does one diagnose and treat flail chest?

Diagnosis: the classic picture of four or more multiply fractured ribs resulting in a flail segment of chest wall that moves **paradoxically** and results in immediate hypoventilation; (a much more common clinical picture is that of multiple rib fractures with underlying pulmonary contusion that results in progressive respiratory failure)
Treatment: **intubation** with positive pressure ventilation and PEEP

How does one diagnose and treat cardiac tamponade?

Diagnosis: **Beck's triad** of decreased heart sounds, jugular venous distention, and decreased blood pressure; also tachycardia, pulsus paradoxus, Kussmaul's sign; hypotension due to tamponade implies imminent cardiac collapse
Treatment: immediate IV fluid bolus, **pericardiocentesis** → subsequent surgical exploration is mandatory

How does one diagnose and treat massive hemothorax?

Diagnosis: hypotension, unilaterally decreased or absent breath sounds, dullness to percussion; obvious on CXR if massive (but remember up to 500 ml of blood can be hidden by the diaphragm on upright CXR)
Treatment: volume replacement, **tube thoracostomy** (chest tube); use a cell saver if available; removal of the blood will allow

apposition of the parietal and visceral pleura, which will seal the defect, slowing the bleeding

CIRCULATION

What are the goals in assessing circulation?

Securing adequate tissue perfusion, treatment of external bleeding

What is the initial test for adequate circulation?

Palpation of pulses; as a rough guide, if a radial pulse is palpable, then systolic pressure is at least 80 mm Hg, and if a femoral or carotid pulse is palpable, then systolic pressure is at least 60 mm Hg

What comprises adequate assessment of circulation?

Heart rate, blood pressure, peripheral perfusion, urinary output, mental status; beware of relying only on the blood pressure: especially in the young, autonomic tone can maintain blood pressure until cardiovascular collapse is imminent, capillary refill (normal <2 seconds), exam of skin: cold, clammy = hypovolemia

How are sites of external bleeding treated?

By direct pressure; avoid tourniquets and blind clamping of bleeding sites, both lead to increased limb loss

What is the preferred intravenous access in the trauma patient?

Two large-bore (14–16 gauge) intravenous catheters in the upper extremities

What are alternate sites of intravenous access?

Percutaneous and cutdown catheters in the lower leg saphenous (cutdown) and femoral veins (percutaneous); avoid subclavian and jugular lines if possible because of their increased morbidity in the trauma patient

How does one remember the anatomy of the right groin for a femoral vein catheter?

NAVEL: N, nerve; A, artery; V, vein; E, extralymphatic material; L, lymphatics; thus, the vein is medial to the femoral artery pulse

What is the resuscitation fluid of choice?

Lactated Ringer's solution; LR is isotonic and the lactate helps buffer the hypovolemia induced metabolic acidosis

What types of decompression must the trauma patient receive?

Gastric decompression with a NG tube and Foley catheter bladder decompression **after normal rectal exam**

How do you get gastric decompression with a maxillofacial fracture?	NOT with a nasogastric tube, as the tube may perforate the cribriform plate and into the brain if maxillofacial fracture/skull fracture; place an **oral**-gastric tube (OGT) not a NG tube

DISABILITY

What are the goals in assessing disability?	Determination of neurologic injury (think, neurologic disability)
What comprises adequate assessment of disability?	Mental status: Glasgow coma scale (GCS) Pupils: a blown pupil reflects ipsilateral brain mass (blood) as the CN III is compressed Motor/sensory: screening exam for extremity movement, sensation

GCS Scoring System?

Eyes?

Eye opening (E)

4—Opens spontaneously
3—Opens to voice (command)
2—Opens to painful stimulus
1—Does not open eyes

Motor?

Motor response (M)

6—Obeys commands
5—Localizes painful stimulus
4—Withdraws from pain
3—Decorticate posture
2—Decerebrate posture
1—No movement

Verbal?

Verbal response (V)

5—Appropriate and oriented
4—Confused
3—Inappropriate words
2—Incomprehensible sounds
1—No sounds

EXPOSURE

What are the goals in obtaining adequate exposure?	Complete disrobing to allow a thorough visual inspection and digital palpation of the patient during the secondary survey

SECONDARY SURVEY

What principle is followed in completing the secondary survey?	Complete physical examination including all orifices: ears, nose, mouth, vagina, rectum

Why look in the ears?	Hemotympanum is a sign of basilar skull fracture, otorrhea is a sign of basilar skull fracture
Examination of what part of the trauma patient's body is often forgotten?	The patient's back—logroll the patient and examine!
What are typical signs of basilar skull fracture?	Raccoon eyes, Battle's sign, clear otorrhea or rhinorrhea, hemotympanum
What sign of an anterior chamber bleeding must not be missed on the eye exam?	Traumatic hyphema
What potentially destructive lesion must not be missed on the nasal exam?	Nasal septal hematoma; the hematoma must be evacuated as if not it will result in pressure necrosis of septum!
What is the best indication of a mandibular fracture?	Dental malocclusion; ask the patient "bite down" and "does that feel normal to you?"
What signs of thoracic trauma are often found on the neck exam?	Crepitus or subcutaneous emphysema from tracheobronchial disruption, tracheal deviation from tension pneumothorax, jugular venous distention from cardiac tamponade, carotid bruit heard with seatbelt neck injury resulting in carotid artery injury
What is the best exam for broken ribs or sternum?	Lateral and anterior-posterior compression of the thorax to elicit pain
What physical signs are diagnostic for thoracic great vessel injury?	None; diagnosis of great vessel injury requires a high index of suspicion based on mechanism of injury, associated injuries, and CXR/radiographic findings
What must be considered in every penetrating injury of the thorax at or below the level of the nipple?	Concomitant injury to the abdomen; remember, the diaphragms go up to the level of the nipples in the male on full expiration
What is the proper technique for examining the thoracic and lumbar spine?	Logrolling the patient to allow complete visualization of the back and palpation of the spine to elicit pain over fxs
What conditions must exist to pronounce an abdominal physical exam negative?	An alert patient without any evidence of head/spinal cord injury or drug/ETOH intoxication
What physical signs may indicate intraabdominal injury?	Guarding, tender, plus rebound tenderness and other signs of peritoneal irritation, progressive distention, absent bowel sounds

What must be documented from the rectal exam?	Sphincter tone as an indication of spinal cord injury; presence of blood as an indication of colon or rectal injury; prostate position as an indication of urethral injury
What is the best technique to test for pelvic and hip fractures?	Lateral compression of the iliac crests and greater trochanters and anterior-posterior compression of the symphysis pubis to elicit pain
What physical signs indicate possible urethral injury, thus contraindicating placement of a Foley catheter?	**High-riding ballotable prostate** on rectal exam, presence of blood at the meatus, scrotal or perineal ecchymosis
What must be documented from the extremity exam?	Any fractures or joint injuries, any open wounds, motor and sensory exam particularly distal to any fractures, distal pulses, and peripheral perfusion
What complication is often seen after prolonged ischemia to an extremity that must be treated immediately to save the extremity, and what is that treatment?	**Compartment syndrome,** treated by four-compartment fasciotomy
What injuries must be suspected in a trauma patient with a progressive decline in mental status?	Epidural hematoma, subdural hematoma, brain swelling with rising intracranial pressure; But one must rule out **hypoxia/ hypotension!**

TRAUMA STUDIES

During evaluation of blunt trauma, radiographic films are usually obtained sometime during the primary survey. What films are required?	Lateral cervical spine film, AP (anterior-to-posterior) chest film, AP pelvis film
Also during the primary survey specimens are sent for laboratory analysis. What specimens are usually sent?	Blood for complete blood count, chemistries, coagulation studies, and **type and crossmatch;** urine for urinalysis; blood is often spun in the emergency department for a quick estimate of hematocrit
What films are required to evaluate for possible cervical spinal injury?	Lateral spine, AP spine, open-mouth odontoid

What vertebral body must be seen to adequately evaluate a lateral cervical spine film?	T-1
What options are there to see this vertebral body beyond the lateral spine film?	Swimmer's view, spine CT scan
What findings on the chest film are suggestive of thoracic great vessel injury?	*Widened mediastinum, first rib fracture, apical pleural capping, loss of aortic contour/KNOB/a-p window, depression of left main stem bronchus, nasogastric tube/tracheal deviation, pleural effusion
What study is used to rule out thoracic great vessel injury?	Thoracic arch aortogram; gold standard
What studies are available to evaluate for intraabdominal injury?	Diagnostic peritoneal lavage (DPL) and CT scan (Laparoscopy and ultrasound are being evaluated for use in trauma diagnosis)
What are the respective advantages of these studies?	Peritoneal lavage (DPL) is a sensitive and specific test for intraperitoneal blood, and can be rapidly completed in the emergency room, operating room, or even in the CT scanner while the head is being studied. But DPL does not evaluate the retroperitoneum! CT scanning can detect retroperitoneal injury and can better localize and characterize an injury, thus giving the option of nonoperative therapy (e.g., liver laceration/spleen laceration). But CT misses small bowel injury.
Name an absolute contraindication to both peritoneal lavage and CT scanning in the evaluation of abdominal trauma.	Obvious need for laparotomy; for example, progressive abdominal distention with hypotension, gunshot wounds to the abdomen, stab wounds to the abdomen with peritoneal signs
How do you do a DPL?	Place a catheter below the umbilicus (in patients without a pelvic fracture) into abdominal cavity and infuse 1 liter of saline or LR; then drain the fluid (by gravity) and analyze the fluid
Where do you place the DPL catheter in a patient with a pelvic fracture?	**Above the umbilicus!** a common error! if you go below the umbilicus you may get into a pelvic hematoma tracking between the fascia layers and thus a false-positive DPL

Indicators of a positive peritoneal lavage?

Lavaged fluid

1. Classic: inability to read newsprint through lavaged fluid
2. RBC > 100,000/mm^3
3. WBC > 500/mm^3 (*Note:* mm^3 NOT mm^2)
4. Lavage fluid (LR/NS) drained from chest tube, Foley, NG tube

Also less common:

5. Bile present
6. Bacteria present
7. Feces present
8. Vegetable matter present
9. Elevated amylase level

What must be in place before one performs a DPL?

NG tube and Foley catheter—to remove the stomach and bladder from the firing line!

What study is used to evaluate the urethra in cases of possible disruption due to blunt trauma?

Retrograde cystourethrogram

What is the most emergent orthopaedic injury?

Hip dislocation—must be reduced immediately (on x-ray table or during resuscitation in ER!)

Define the anatomy of neck by trauma zones:

Zone III?

Angle of the mandible and up

Zone II?

Angle of the mandible to the cricoid cartilage

Zone I?

Below the cricoid cartilage
(Think of the zone Roman numerals piled in anatomic order: III
                                                                  II
                                                                  I

and thus, forming the shape of a face. *Note:* the zones are in the same anatomic order as the LeFort facial fractures III, II, I!)

How do you Rx penetrating (that penetrate the platysma) neck injuries by neck zone

Zone III?

A-gram first

Zone II?

Surgical exploration

Zone I?

A-gram first

What films are typically obtained to evaluate extremity fractures?	Complete views of the involved extremity including the joints above and below the fracture

MISCELLANEOUS TRAUMA FACTS

What is the "3 for 1" rule?	The trauma patient in hypovolemic shock acutely requires 3 ml of crystalloid (LR) for every 1 ml of blood loss
What is the minimal UO for an adult trauma patient?	50 ml/hr
Findings that would require a celiotomy in a blunt trauma victim?	Peritoneal signs, free air on AXR, positive DPL, massive injury on CT scan
Rx for a gunshot wound to the belly?	**Exploratory laparotomy**
Rx for a stab wound to the belly?	If peritoneal signs, lots of bleeding, shock, omentum or bowel sticking out the wound, unstable vital signs, then exploratory laparotomy; otherwise, many surgeons observe the asymptomatic stab wound patient **closely!**
Positive peritoneal tap?	Prior to starting a peritoneal lavage the DPL catheter should be aspirated; if >5 ml of blood or enteric contents are aspirated then this constitutes a positive tap and requires laparotomy
How much blood can be lost into the thigh with a closed femur fracture?	Up to 3 liters of blood or >½ the patient's blood volume!
Can an adult lose enough blood in the skull from a brain injury to cause hypovolemic shock?	Absolutely **NOT!** but INFANTS can lose enough blood from a brain injury to cause shock
What is the brief A.T.L.S. Hx?	An "Ample" Hx: A: allergies M: medications P: PMH L: last meal (when) E: Events (of injury, etc.)
In what population is a surgical cricothyroidotomy not recommended?	Any patient <12 years old; instead perform needle cricothyroidotomy

Rx for subcutaneous emphysema?

Nothing (unless there is external compression by the emphysema of the upper airway—rare)

What is a massive hemothorax?

>1500 ml of blood from the chest tube (Rx initially by IVF and chest tube

Signs of a laryngeal fracture?

1. Subcutaneous emphysema in neck
2. Altered voice
3. Palpable laryngeal fracture

Rx of rectal penetrating injury?

Diverting proximal colostomy, closure of perforation if possible and definitely if intraperitoneal, and **presacral drainage!**

Rx for extraperitoneal minor bladder rupture?

Many use conservative Rx of catheter bladder drainage and observation; intraperitoneal or large bladder rupture requires operative closure in three layers

Intraabdominal injury associated with seatbelt use?

Intestinal injuries, (L2 fx, pancreatic injury)

Rx for pelvic fx?

±MAST trousers until external fixator placed, IVF/blood, SUPRAUMBILICAL DPL, and A-gram to embolize bleeding pelvic vessels; do not enter pelvic hematoma in OR for positive DPL unless major arterial injury

21
Burns

What consideration besides temperature affects the severity of thermal burns?

Heat capacity; moist heat has a much higher heat capacity, and thus capacity to burn, than dry heat

Are acid or alkali chemical burns more serious?

In general, alkali burns because the body cannot buffer the alkali, thus allowing them to burn for much longer

Why are electrical burns so dangerous?

Most of the destruction from electrical burns is internal, as the route of least electrical resistance follows nerves, blood vessels, and fascia. Injury is usually far worse than external burns at entrance and exit sites would indicate. **Cardiac arrhythmias,** myoglobinuria, acidosis, and renal failure are common.

How do you treat myoglobinuria?

To avoid renal injury:
1. Hydrate with IV fluids
2. Mannitol diuresis
3. Alkalize urine with IV bicarbonate

First degree burns involve which skin structures?

Epidermis only

How do they present?

Painful, dry, red areas that do not form blisters; think "**sunburn**"

Second degree burns involve which skin structures?

Epidermis and varying levels of dermis

How do they present?

Painful, hypersensitive, swollen, mottled areas with blisters and open weeping surfaces

Third degree burns involve which skin structures?

All layers of the skin including skin appendages, blood vessels, and nerve endings

How do they present?

Painless, insensate, swollen, dry, mottled white, and charred areas

Burn severity is determined by which measure?

The total body surface area (TBSA) affected by second and third degree burns; TBSA is calculated by the "rule of nines" in adults and by a modified rule in children to account for the disproportionate size of the head and trunk

What is the "rule of nines"?

In an adult, the total body surface area that is burned can be estimated by the following:
Each upper limb = 9%
Each lower limb = 18%
Ant. + post. trunk = 18% each
Head and neck = 9%
Perineum and genitalia = 1%

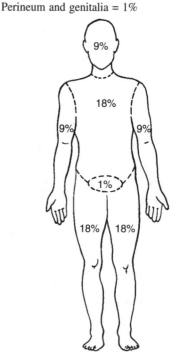

What technique can be used to estimate TBSA in small or discontinuous burns?

The "rule of the palm": the surface area of the palm is approximately 1% of the TBSA

What are the hospitalization criteria for burn patients?

1. Second degree burns greater than 20% TBSA
2. Third degree burns greater than 10% TBSA
3. Any burns greater than 10% TBSA in children and the elderly

4. Any burns involving the face, hands, feet, or perineum
5. Any burns with inhalation injury
6. Any burns with associated trauma
7. Any electrical burns

What is the first treatment step for any burn?

Stop the burning process; immediately remove all clothes, remove hot and adherent substances such as grease and tar, and copiously irrigate all chemical burns with water; chemical eye burns require prolonged (up to 8 hours) flushing

Once this is accomplished, what principles guide the assessment and resuscitation of the burn patient?

Airway, breathing, circulation, disability, and exposure, as for the trauma patient

Signs of smoke inhalation?

Smoke and soot in sputum/mouth/nose; nasal/facial hair burns, carboxyhemoglobin, throat/mouth erythema, hx of L.O.C. (loss of consciousness)/explosion/fire in small enclosed area, dyspnea, low O_2 saturation

How should the airway be managed in the burn patient with an inhalational injury?

With a low threshold for **intubation;** oropharyngeal swelling may so occlude the airway that intubation is impossible, either very rapidly or slowly and progressively over 24–48 hours; 100% oxygen should be administered immediately and continued until significant carboxyhemoglobin is ruled out

What is the "Parkland formula"?

Formula widely used to estimate the volume (V) of crystalloid necessary for the initial resuscitation of the burn patient; half of the calculated volume is given in the **first 8 hours,** the rest in the next 16 hours

$$V = TBSA\ (\%) \times Wgt\ (kg) \times 4$$

KNOW THIS FORMULA!

How is the crystalloid given?

Through two large-bore peripheral venous catheters introduced through unburned skin

What fluid is used after the first 24–36 hours postburn?

Initially **crystalloid** is used as the capillaries leak! but after 24–36 hours the capillaries begin to work and then the patient can usually benefit from **albumin** IV (A.K.A. colloid)

How is volume status monitored in the burn patient?

Blood pressure, heart rate, peripheral perfusion, mental status, and **urinary output;** Foley catheter is mandatory, and may be supplemented by central venous pressure and pulmonary capillary pressure monitoring

Why is it important to monitor temperature closely in the burn patient?

Temperature tends to be very labile due to exposure, fluid losses with evaporation, administration of large volumes of hypothermic fluids, and central temperature instability; hypothermia predisposes to cardiac irritability and coagulopathy

Why do most severely burned patients require nasogastric decompression?

Patients with greater than 20% TBSA burns usually develop a paralytic **ileus** → VOMITING → ASPIRATION RISK → PNEUMONIA

How are minor burns dressed?

Minor burns are treated initially with cold compresses for pain relief. After gentle cleaning with nonionic detergent and debridement of loose skin and broken blisters, the burn is dressed with a topical antibacterial (silver sulfadiazine, neomycin) and covered with a sterile dressing.

Note some advantages and disadvantages of each.

1. **Silver nitrate**—broad spectrum, painless and inexpensive, but nonpenetrating and may cause **electrolyte imbalances**
2. **Silver sulfadiazine**—painless, no electrolyte imbalances, no need for occlusive dressing, but little penetration, misses *Pseudomonas,* and has idiosyncratic **neutropenia;** agent of choice for small burns
3. **Mafenide**—penetrates eschars, broad spectrum (but misses *Staphylococcus*), but pain and burning on application; allergic reaction in 7%; may cause **acid-base imbalances;** agent of choice in already contaminated burn wounds

How are major burns dressed?

Following only gentle cleaning the burns are dressed with topical antibiotic and sterile dressings; cold compresses are avoided. Gentle debridement through dressing changes and over several days will allow second degree burns to heal and will prepare third degree burns for grafting.

Are prophylactic systemic antibiotics administered to burn patients?

No. Prophylactic antibiotics have not been shown to reduce the incidence of sepsis, but rather have been shown to select for resistant organisms

Circumferential, full-thickness burns to the extremities are at risk for what complication?

Distal neurovascular impairment similar to compartment syndrome

How is it treated?

Escharotomy: full-thickness longitudinal incision through the eschar with scalpel or electrocautery; incision must extend into healthy fat

Is tetanus prophylaxis required in the burn patient?

Yes, mandatory in all patients except those actively immunized within the past 12 months

What is the most common fault in the care of burn patients?

Delay in treatment; many complications of severe burns, including renal failure and sepsis, are severely aggravated by inadequate or delayed fluid resuscitation

Water evaporation is highest from which burns?

3rd degree

Can infection convert a split-thickness injury into a full-thickness injury?

Yes!

Most common burn wound bacteria?

Pseudomonas

How does one Rx carbon monoxide inhalation overdose?

100% O_2

What electrolyte must be followed very closely acutely after a burn?

Na^+

22
Upper GI Bleeding

Symptoms?	(Possible) hematemesis, melena, syncope, shock Sx, fatigue, coffee-ground emesis, hematochezia, epigastric discomfort
Why hematochezia?	Blood is a cathartic
Signs?	Signs of hypotension, + Hemoccult
Risk factors?	ETOH, cigarettes, liver disease, burn/trauma, aspirin/NSAIDs, vomiting, sepsis, steroids, previous bleeding, hx of PUD/esophageal varices, splenic vein thrombosis, etc.
Causes? (by % occurrence)	Peptic ulcer disease: **duodenal ulcer** (25%), **gastric ulcer** (20%) *Note:* PUD about 50%, **acute gastritis** (20%), esophageal varices (20%), Mallory-Weiss tear (10%), others (<5%): gastric CA, esophagitis, pancreatitis, hemobilia, duodenal diverticula, gastric volvulus, Boerhaave's, aortoenteric fistula, paraesophageal hiatal hernia, epistaxis, NG tube irritation
Diagnostic tests?	History, NG tube aspirate, EGD (endoscopy), abdominal x-ray˜
Lab tests?	Chem-7, bili, LFTs, CBC, **type & cross,** PT/PTT, amylase
Why elevated BUN?	Because of absorption of blood by the GI tract
Initial treatment?	1. IVFs (16G or larger peripheral IVs × 2), Foley catheter (monitor fluid status) 2. NG suction (determine rate & amount of blood)

3. Water lavage (use warm H_2O—will remove clots, facilitating EGD (esophagogastroduodenoscopy)
4. EGD: Endoscopy (determine etiology/ location of bleed and possible treatment—coagulate bleeders)

Indications for surgical interventional in UGI bleeding?

Profuse bleeding with hypotension, recurrent bleeding

Percentage needing surgery?

About 20%

Percentage spontaneously stop bleeding?

85% stop bleeding within a few hours of admission

Percentage rebleeding after admission?

25%

Mortality of initial bleeding?

<5%

Mortality of rebleeding?

About $\frac{1}{3}$

PEPTIC ULCER DISEASE

What is it?

Includes gastric & duodenal ulcers

Incidence in U.S.?

Approx. 10% of all Americans will suffer from PUD during their lifetime!

Consequences of PUD?

Pain, hemorrhage, perforation, obstruction

Bacteria associated with PUD?

Helicobacter pylori (Rx with bismuth)

DUODENAL ULCER

Mean age?

20–40 y.o., M > F (young)

Incidence?

More common than gastric ulcer

Location?

Majority are within 2 cm of pylorus in duodenal bulb

Cause?

Due to **increased gastric acid** production

Risks?   Smoking, uremia, Z-E syndrome

Symptoms?   Epigastric pain—burning or aching,
                                    usually several hours after a meal, pain
                                    is relieved by food, milk, or antacids,
                                    may also c/o back pain (indicating
                                    ulcer into pancreas), N/V, anorexia,
                                    ↓ appetite.

Signs?   ± Tenderness in epigastric area, guaiac +,
                                    melena, hematochezia

DDx?   Acute abdomen, pancreatitis, cholecystitis,
                                    Z-E, gastritis, MI, gastric ulcer

Diagnosis?   History, PE, EGD, UGI series

Prevention?   Avoid aspirin, nicotine, alcohol, reserpine,
                                    caffeine/other xanthines

Medical treatment?   **H2 receptor antagonists**—(H2 blockers)
                                    heal ulcer in 4–6 weeks in majority;
                                    antacids—to control gastric pH, promote
                                    healing; **sucralfate**—coats ulcer;
                                    omeprazole—(↓ acid production by
                                    stopping H^+-K^+ ion pump) use for
                                    refractory ulcers and ulcers associated
                                    with Z-E

When is surgery indicated?   1. Fail medical Rx (intractability)
                                    2. Massive bleeding
                                    3. Perforation
                                    4. Obstruction (gastric outlet obstruction)

Goal of surgery?   Decrease gastric acid secretion

TYPES OF SURGERIES _____

   Vagotomy (define)   Truncal vagotomy: resect 1–2 cm segment of
                                    each vagal trunk as it enters abdomen on
                                    distal esophogus—this decreases gastric acid
                                    secretion **and** gastric emptying; also selective
                                    vagotomies

If you do truncal vagotomy, what else must you do?

A **drainage procedure** (pyloroplasty, antrectomy, or gastrojejunostomy), since vagal fibers provide relaxation of the pylorus and if you cut them the pylorus will not open

Advantage of proximal gastric vagotomy (highly selective vagotomy)?

No drainage procedure needed; vagal fibers to pylorus are preserved, low rate of dumping syndrome.
Proximal **g**astric **v**agotomy; (PGV)

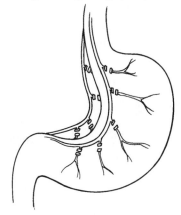

Vagotomy & pyloroplasty?

Do a pyloroplasty to compensate for decreased gastric emptying with vagotomy

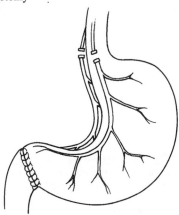

Vagotomy & antrectomy: Remove antrum in addition to
                              vagotomy—reconstruct as Billroth I or
                              Billroth II

                              Billroth I:

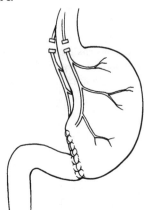

                              Billroth II:

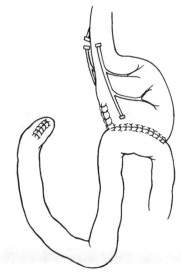

Which ulcer operation has the   PGV (proximal gastric vagotomy)
***highest* ulcer recurrence rate**
and the *lowest* dumping rate?

Which ulcer operation has the   Vagotomy and antrectomy
***lowest* ulcer recurrence rate**
and the *highest* dumping rate?

Why may a duodenal rupture be painless?

Fluid can be sterile with a nonirritating pH of 7.0

Why may a perforated duodenal ulcer present as lower quadrant abdominal pain?

Fluid from stomach/bile drains down paracolic gutters to lower quadrants and causes localized irritation

GASTRIC ULCER

Mean age?

40–70 y.o. (older)

Location?

95% are on lesser curvature, with 60% of these within 6 cm of pylorus

Cause?

Ulcer is due to **decreased cytoprotection** or gastric protection (i.e., decreased mucous production)

Is gastric acid production high or low?

Nl or low gastric acid production

Risks?

Smoking, ETOH, burns, trauma, CNS tumor/trauma, NSAIDs, steroids, shock, severe illness

Symptoms?

Pain—transiently relieved by food/antacids; pain recurs usually within 30 min of eating; attacks are long; vomiting, anorexia, aggrevation of pain with eating, chronicity, wt loss

Diagnosis?

History, PE, EGD with multiple Bx

When/why biopsy?

With all gastric ulcers *must* rule out gastric cancer. If the ulcer does not heal in 6 weeks after medical Rx must rebiopsy (biopsy in OR also)

Medical treatment?

Similar to that of duodenal ulcer (H2 blockers, etc.)

Indications for surgery?

1. Hemorrhage
2. Perforation
3. Obstruction
4. Intractibility

Common operation?

Distal gastrectomy with excision of the ulcer *without* vagotomy unless duodenal DZ

Recurrence rate?

$\approx \frac{2}{3}$ in 2 years with medical treatment alone, usually recur within 6 months of first event

Define _____

Cushing's ulcer	PUD/gastritis associated with **CNS** trauma or tumor (think, Dr. Cushing = neurosurgeon)
Curling's ulcer	PUD/gastritis associated with major **burn** injury

PERFORATED PEPTIC ULCER

Symptoms?	Acute onset of upper abdominal pain, or in lower quadrants, may be diffuse pain
Why pain in lower quadrants?	From passage of perforated fluid along colic gutters
Signs?	Decreased BS, tympanic sound over liver (air), peritoneal signs, tender abdomen
Sign of post. erosion?	Bleeding from gastroduodenal artery (and acute pancreatitis)
Sign of ant. perf?	Free air (anterior more common than posterior perf)
DDx?	Acute pancreatitis, acute cholecystitis, perforated acute appendicitis, colonic diverticulitis, MI, any perforated viscus
Diagnostic tests?	X-ray: free air under diaphragm or in lesser sac in upright CXR (if upright CXR not possible, then left lateral decubitus, as air can be seen over liver and not confused with gastric bubble), peritoneal lavage in obtunded patient Exploratory laporatomy
Lab findings?	Mild leukocytosis, high amylase in peritoneal fluid/**serum** (secondary to absorption into blood stream from peritoneum)
Initial treatment?	1. NG tube—↓ contamination of peritoneal cavity 2. Antibiotics 3. Surgery—close perf ± ulcer operation (e.g., vagotomy and pyloroplasty), irrigation of peritoneal cavity
What is a Graham patch?	A piece of omentum incorporated into suture closure
Mortality?	About 10%
Increased mortality associated with?	↑ Age, female sex, gastric perforation

Significance of hemorrhage and perforation?	May signify 2 ulcers (kissing), post. is bleeding and ant. is perforated with free air
Late complications after ulcer surgery?	Recurrent ulcer (marginal ulcer common), dumping syndrome, vitamin deficiency

MALLORY-WEISS SYNDROME

What is it?	Post-retching longitudinal tear (submucosa & mucosa) of the stomach near GE junction; about $\frac{3}{4}$ in stomach
Causes of tear?	Increased gastric pressure, often aggravated by hiatal hernia
Risk factors?	Retching, alcoholic ($\frac{1}{2}$), >50% have hiatal hernia
Symptoms?	Epigastric pain, thoracic substernal pain
Signs?	Post-retching hematemesis
Diagnosis?	History, PE, EGD
"Classic" history?	First vomit food & gastric contents, followed by forceful retching and then bloody vomitus
Treatment?	Room temp. water lavage (90% stop bleeding), electrocautery, arterial embolization, surgery for refractory bleeding

BOERHAAVE'S SYNDROME

What is it?	Postemetic esophogeal rupture (all layers), doesn't bleed profusely very frequently
Location?	Most often in posterolateral aspect of esophogus (on left), 3–5 cm above GE jxn
Cause of rupture?	Increased intraluminal pressure, usually caused by violent retching and vomiting
Symptoms?	Pain postemesis—may radiate to back, dysphagia
Signs?	L pneumothorax (but may be rt-sided), Hamman's sign, L pleural effusion, subcutaneous/mediastinal emphysema, fever, tachypnea, tachycardia, signs of infx by 24 hr, neck crepitus
What is Hamman's sign?	"Mediastinal crunch"—produced by the heart beating against air-filled tissues

Diagnosis	History, PE, CXR, esophogram with water-soluble contrast
Treatment?	Surgery within 24 hr to drain the mediastinum and surgically close the perforation; broad-spectrum antibiotics

GASTRIC CANCER

Incidence?	Rare in U.S. (higher in Japan)
Risks?	**Diet:** smoked meats, high nitrates, low fruits & veggies, ETOH, tobacco **Environment:** raised in high-risk area, poor socioeconomic status
Mean age?	>60 y.o. at discovery
M:F ratio?	2:1
Symptoms?	Possible: postprandial, epigastric pain/discomfort, anorexia/wgt loss, dysphagia, hematemesis, melena
Signs?	Anemia, melena, heme occult, epigastric mass, hepatomegaly, coffee-ground emesis, Blumer's shelf, Virchow node, enlarged ovaries
What is a Blumer shelf?	A solid peritoneal deposit anterior to the rectum, forming a "shelf," palpated on **rectal examination**
What is a Virchow node?	Metastatic gastric CA to nodes in neck, specifically **L supraclavicular** fossa
What is Sister Mary Joseph's sign?	Periumbilical lymph node gastric CA mets—presents as **periumbilical mass**
What is a Krukenburg tumor?	Gastric CA (or other adeno CA) that has metastasized to the ovary—enlarged ovaries
Diagnostic tests?	UGI series, EGD, biopsy all gastric ulcers at operation and at EGD
Histology?	Majority are adenocarcinoma
Morphology?	1. Ulcerative ($\frac{1}{4}$)—ulcer through all layers 2. Polyploid ($\frac{1}{4}$) 3. Superficial spreading ($\frac{1}{10}$)—early cancer, through mucosa/submucosa

4. Linitis plastica ($\frac{1}{10}$)—"leather bottle" due to early spread through all layers
5. Advanced cancer—part within and part beyond stomach

Treatment?

Surgical resection with wide (6 cm) margins (total or subtotal gastrectomy), ± chemo, lymph node dissection

When do a splenectomy?

Most would do a splenectomy during resection for gastric cancer when the tumor directly invades the spleen/splenic hilum, or with splenic hilar adenopathy

Stages/Prognosis _____

I?

To submucosa; $\frac{2}{3}$ 5-yr survival

II?

To muscularis propria; $\frac{1}{3}$ 5-yr survival

III?

Positive lymph nodes without distant mets; 10% 5-yr survival

IV?

Positive lymph nodes **and** distant mets or contiguous spread; basically 0% 5-yr survival (Think, gastric CA stages I, II, III, IV corresponds **roughly** to colorectal Duke's stages A, B, C, D, respectively)

Percentage that have mets at Dx?

About $\frac{3}{4}$

Location of cancer in stomach?

40% in antrum, mainly lesser curvature, (as seen with benign gastric ulcer); 30% in body & fundus

23
Small Intestine and Appendicitis

SMALL BOWEL OBSTRUCTION

What is it?

Mechanical occlusion of the bowel lumen (mechanical obstruction) or paralysis of intestinal musculature (paralytic ileus) resulting in accumulation of fluid and gas proximal to the obstruction and distention of the bowel wall

What are the physiologic changes that occur with an obstruction?

Distention results in decreased absorption (lumen-to-blood) and increased secretion (blood-to-lumen), thereby leading to further distention as well as fluid and electrolyte abnormalities. Bacterial proliferation occurs due to stasis; but, this probably has no role in the clinical picture of simple mechanical obstruction, since the bacteria or bacterial toxins do not cross normal intestinal lumen acutely.

What are the causes?

Mechanical obstruction: obstruction of the lumen—polypoid tumors, intussusception, gallstone ileus, impacted feces or meconium, bezoar

Intrinsic lesions of the bowel—congenital, neoplastic, inflammatory, or iatrogenic strictures

Extrinsic lesions of the bowel—postoperative adhesions, inflammation, hernias, neoplastic masses, abscesses, volvulus

Common mimic?

Paralytic ileus—a common disorder occurring in most patients undergoing abdominal surgery; caused by a combination of neural, humoral, and metabolic factors; also seen with inflammatory processes in the abdomen such as pancreatitis, peritonitis

How are SBOs commonly categorized?

Partial vs. complete; partial obstruction, depending on the cause is often managed conservatively (i.e., without surgery) since the risk of ischemic necrosis is much less than with complete obstruction; operative intervention is required for complete obstruction

What is the #1 adult cause?

Postoperative **adhesions!

Common causes of SBO in adults?

Adhesions, hernias, tumors

What is the #1 pediatric cause?

**Hernias!

Clinical presentation?

Crampy, paroxysmal abdominal pain (colic), **vomiting,** obstipation, abdominal **distention,** and failure to pass flatus (although flatus may still be present), **high-pitched bowel sounds** separated by relatively quiet periods; tachycardia and hypotension in relation to the degree of hypovolemia

Radiographic presentation?

Distended bowel proximal to the obstruction, **air-fluid levels,** foreign bodies

Radiology test to differentiate partial from complete SBO?

Contrast study from above = **enteroclysis**

Management?

Initially, **IV fluid,** electrolyte and acid/base correction, **NG decompression**
If obstruction does not resolve, timing of surgery depends on

1. The duration of the obstruction, i.e., severity of fluid, electrolyte, and acid/base abnormalities
2. The need to improve vital organ function prior to surgery
3. The risk of strangulation

Signs of strangulated bowel?

Fever, severe/continuous pain, hemetemesis, **shock,** gas in the bowel wall or portal vein, abdominal free air, **peritoneal signs, acidosis** (increased lactic acid)

Clinical parameters that will lower the threshold to operate on a SBO?

1. Increasing **WBC**
2. **Fever**
3. **Tachycardia**
4. **Peritoneal signs,** particularly if localizing

SMALL BOWEL TUMORS

DDx of benign tumors of the small intestine?	Leiomyoma, lipoma, lymphangioma, fibroma, adenomas, hemangiomas
Most common benign small bowel tumor?	**Leiomyoma**
DDx of malignant tumors of the small intestine?	Adenocarcinoma, carcinoid, lymphoma
Most common malignant small bowel tumor?	**Adenocarcinoma**

MECKEL'S DIVERTICULUM

What is it?	**Remnant of the omphalomesenteric duct/ vitelline duct,** which connects the yolk sac with the primitive midgut in the embryo
Usual location?	Within about 2 feet of the ileocecal valve on the **antimesenteric** border of the bowel
Major differential diagnosis?	*Appendicitis*
Is it a true diverticulum?	**Yes,** all layers of the intestine are found in the wall
Incidence?	About 2% of the population at autopsy, but >90% of these are asymptomatic
Sex ratio?	3× more common in **males**
Age at onset of sx?	Most frequently in the first **two years of life,** but can occur at any age
Complications?	*Intestinal hemorrhage* (painless)—50%; accounts for half of all lower GI bleeding in patients <2 y.o. bleeding due to ectopic gastric mucosa secreting acid → ulcer → bleeding *Intestinal obstruction*—25%; most common complication in adults; includes volvulus and intussusception *Inflammation* (±perforation)—20%
Heterotopic tissue?	Present in >50% of cases; usually (85%) is **gastric mucosa,** but duodenal, pancreatic, and colonic
Rule of "2s"?	—2% are **symptomatic** —Found about **2 feet** from the ileocecal valve —Found in 2% of the population

What is a Meckel's scan?

Scan for ectopic gastric mucosa in Meckel's diverticulum; uses **technetium pertechnetate** IV, which is preferentially taken up by gastric mucosa

APPENDICITIS

What is it?

Obstruction of the appendiceal lumen producing a closed loop with resultant inflammation that can lead to necrosis and perforation

Causes?

Fecalith (A.K.A. appendolith), **lymphoid hyperplasia,** parasite, foreign body

Presentation?

Onset of referred or periumbilical pain followed by anorexia, nausea, and vomiting; *Note:* unlike gastroenteritis, *pain precedes vomiting;* pain then migrates to the RLQ where it becomes more intense and localized due to local peritoneal irritation; the presentation may vary depending on the anatomical location of the appendix. *If the patient is hungry and can eat—seriously question the diagnosis of appendicitis

Dx?

History and physical exam

Signs/Sx?

Signs of peritoneal irritation may be present—guarding, muscle spasm, rebound tenderness, obturator and psoas signs, low-grade fever rising to high-grade if perforation occurs

Differential Dx?

Intussusception, volvulus, Meckel's diverticulum, Crohn's disease, ovarian torsion, cyst, or tumor, perforated ulcer, pancreatitis, PID, ruptured ectopic pregnancy, mesenteric lymphadenitis, mittelschmerz

Labs?

—Increased WBC (>10,000 per mm^3 in >90% of cases)
—UA to rule out pyelonephritis or renal calculus
**Mild hematuria and pyuria are *very* common in appendicitis with pelvic inflammation

What is the "hamburger" sign?	Ask patients with suspected appendicitis if they would like a hamburger or their favorite food—if they can really eat, seriously question the diagnosis
Radiographic studies?	CXR to R/O RML or RLL pneumonia, abdominal films usually nonspecific, but calcified fecalith present in about 5%
Rx?	If not perforated—prompt appy + cefoxitin avoids perforation; if perforated—triple abx, fluid resuscitation and prompt appendectomy; all pus is drained and cultures obtained, with postop abx continued for 5–7 days; wound left open in most cases of perforation after closing fascia (heals by secondary intention or delayed primary)
Rx appendiceal abscess?	Most drain abscess/antibx, followed by elective appendectomy ≈6–8 weeks later
If one finds a normal appendix upon exploration, what must one exam/rule out?	Meckel's diverticulum, Crohn's disease, intussusception, gyn causes (ovarian cysts, etc.)
Risk of perforation?	≈25% after 24 hr from onset of Sx ≈50% by 36 hr ≈75% by 48 hr

Define: _____

Mittelschmerz	Lower quadrant pain due to ovulation
Obturator sign	Pain upon internal rotation of the leg with the hip and knee flexed; seen in patients with appendicitis/pelvic abscess
Psoas sign	Pain elicited by extending the hip with the knee in full extension; seen with appendicitis and psoas inflammation
Rovsing's sign	Palpation of the LLQ results in pain in the RLQ; seen in appendicitis

APPENDICEAL TUMORS

Most common appendiceal tumor?	Carcinoid tumor
DDx of appendiceal tumor?	Carcinoid, adenocarcinoma, malignant mucoid adenocarcinoma

In the patient with guaiac + stool and a negative upper and lower GI w/u—what must be ruled out?

A small bowel tumor! evaluate with an enteroclysis (small bowel contrast study)

Most common general surgical abdominal emergency in pregnancy?

Appendicitis (about 1/1750)—due to enlarged uterus appendix may be in the RUQ!

Complications of appendicitis/ appendectomy?

Abscess, free perforation, hepatic abscess, wound infection, appendiceal stump abscess, wound/inguinal hernia, minor bleeding, portal pyelothrombophlebitis (very RARE!)

What percentage of the population has a retrocecal appendix?

About 15%

24
Carcinoid Tumors

What is it?

Tumor arising from neuroendocrine cells (APUDomas) A.K.A. **Kulchitsky cells;** basically, a tumor that secretes **serotonin**

Incidence?

ABOUT ¼ OF ALL SMALL BOWEL TUMORS!

Common sites of occurrence?

Appendix most common site! then ileum *Note:* >80% occur in the GI tract, but they can arise elsewhere (i.e., the **bronchus**)

Signs/Sx?

Depends on the location, with most being asymptomatic; also can present with small bowel obstruction, abdominal pain, bleeding, weight loss, intussusception, or the carcinoid syndrome

What is the carcinoid syndrome?

*Cutaneous flushing, diarrhea, rt-sided heart failure (due to valve failure), bronchospasm;** present in approximately ¹⁄₁₀ of cases and occurs most frequently in midgut tumors; rarely occurs with hindgut tumors (i.e., rectal CA); symptoms result from excessive **serotonin** production by the tumor

Why does the carcinoid syndrome happen in some tumors and not others?

It occurs when **venous drainage from the tumor gains access to the systemic circulation** (i.e., the serotonin and other vasoactive substances escape hepatic degradation) in the following scenarios:

1. Liver metastases
2. Retroperitoneal disease draining into paravertebral veins
3. Primary tumor outside the GI tract and/or portal venous drainage (e.g., ovary, bronchus)

What does the liver break down the serotonin to?

5-HIAA, 5-hydroxyindoleacetic acid

Diagnostic testing?

Urine 5-HIAA (hydroxyindoleacetic acid) elevated as well as urine and platelet serotonin levels; 5-HIAA is elevated in >50% of cases; also barium enema, upper GI series with small bowel follow-through, and enteroclysis (barium instilled into the intestine via a tube from above for a better evaluation of the small bowel. *Note:* abdominal CT usually not helpful as tumors are small and slow growing, often found on exploratory laparotomy!

Treatment?

Excision of the primary tumor and single or feasible mets in the liver; chemotherapy for advanced disease; medical therapy for palliation of the carcinoid syndrome (serotonin antagonists, somatostatin analogue—Octreotide
Octreotide has been shown to relieve diarrhea and flushing in >¾ of cases

Prognosis?

⅔ alive at 5 yr if localized disease
⅓ alive after 5 years if mets

What does carcinoid tumor look like?

Usually intramural bowel mass; cut open—**YELLOW**ish tumor

When is a rt hemicolectomy indicated versus appendectomy for appendiceal carcinoid?

If the tumor is **more than 2 cm,** rt **hemicolectomy** is indicated; if no signs of serosal involvement and **<2 cm, appendectomy**

25
Fistulas

What is a fistula?

An abnormal **communication** between two hollow organs or a hollow organ and the exterior

Predisposing factors and conditions that maintain patency of the fistula?

The acronym "FRIEND" is helpful:

Foreign body
Radiation
Infection
Epithelization
Neoplasm
Distal obstruction

Note: not increased flow—and steroids may inhibit closure but will usually not maintain fistula

SPECIFIC TYPES OF FISTULAS

Enterocutaneous?

Fistula discharging through the abdominal wall, which can occur following GI surgery (anastomotic leak), trauma, or Crohn's disease; complications include high-output fistulas leading to malnutrition and skin problems; enterocultaneous = *bowel* to *skin*

Colonic Fistulas?

Include colovesical, colocutaneous, colovaginal, and coloenteric fistulas

Common cause?

Common causes include **diverticulitis** (commonly involve the sigmoid, as 90% of the diverticulitis cases occur here), granulomatous colitis, cancer, IBD, foreign body, and irradiation

Common site?

Most common type is the **colovesical fistula,** which often presents with recurrent UTIs; other signs include pneumaturia, dysuria, and fecaluria; Dx via BE and cystoscopy

Rx?

Rx is surgical with a segmental colon resection and primary anastomosis, and repair/resection of the involved organ

Biliary Fistulas?	Types include biliary-cutaneous (which often presents with bile peritonitis or an external bile leak), biliary-intestinal (see gallstone ileus), and biliary-pleurobronchial (which presents with bile tinged sputum—biloptysis)
Causes?	Common causes include gallstones, PUD, trauma, and neoplasms with sx of extrabiliary accumulation of bile
Gastrocolic Fistulas?	Common causes include penetrating ulcers, **gastric** or **colonic CA** and Crohn's disease
Complications?	Complications include malnutrition, and severe **enteritis** due to reflux of colonic contents into the stomach and small bowel with subsequent bacterial overgrowth
Anorectal Fistulas?	Often present as acute abscesses; most commonly course in the intersphincteric space between the two groups of sphincters and the fat of the ischiorectal fossa directly to the perineal skin; presents as a painful mass near the anus
What is Goodsall's rule?	Fistulas originating **anterior** to a transverse line through the anus will course **straight** ahead and exit anteriorly, while those exiting **posteriorly** have a **curved** tract

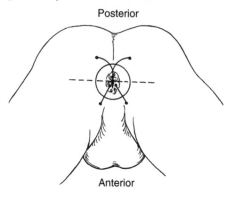

Posterior

Anterior

Management of anorectal fistulas?	1. Define the pathoanatomy 2. Marsupalization of fistula tract (i.e., fillet tract open) 3. Wound care—routine Sitz baths and dressing changes

Pancreatic Enteric Fistula? _____

What is it?

Decompression of a **pseudocyst** or **abscess** into an adjacent organ (a **rare** complication)

Bladder Fistulas? _____

Specific types?

Vesicoenteric (50% due to sigmoid diverticulitis)

Vesicovaginal (most are secondary to gynecological procedures; signs include urinary leak through the vagina, and it is diagnosed by IVP or instilling the bladder with methylene blue and monitoring the vagina for the appearance of dye

Rx?

Surgery involving:

1. Total separation of tissues
2. Sharp excision of fistula tract
3. Closure of defects with absorbable suture without overlapping suture lines
4. Placement of alternative tissues between suture lines if possible (e.g., omentum)

Colon, Rectum, and Anus

COLORECTAL CARCINOMA

What is it?
95% of all colorectal CAs are **adenocarcinomas;** other CAs include carcinoids, lymphomas

What is the incidence?
Most common visceral CA; third most common cause of CA death in men behind lung and prostate and third most common cause of CA death in women behind lung and breast; incidence increases with age starting at age 40 and peaks at 70–80 years; rectal CA contributes 20–30% of all colorectal CA

What is the etiology?
Dietary: low-fiber, high-fat diets correlate with increased rates
Genetic: family history is crucial in history taking

Signs/Sx? _____

Right-sided lesions?
Right side of bowel has large luminal diameter, so tumor may attain large size before diagnosis; chronic fatigue associated with MCHC anemia, occult > gross blood, postprandial discomfort, right-sided mass; obstruction and change in bowel habits uncommon, but may see liquid stools/ electrolyte losses

Left-sided?
Left side of bowel has smaller lumen and semisolid contents; will see change in bowel habits (small-caliber stools), signs of obstruction, abdominal mass, heme(+) or gross blood ± small clots; bleeding rarely massive, constipation

Rectal?
20–30% of all colorectal CA; most common symptom is hematochezia (or passage of red blood ± stool) or — mucus; also tenesmus,

feeling of incomplete evacuation of stool (due to MASS), rectal mass. IMPORTANT: In female patients—vaginal and rectovaginal exam should be included

What are helpful diagnostic tests?

History and physical (*Note:* **approximately 10% of cancers are palpable**), heme occult, CBC, barium enema, sigmoid/colonscopy; *Remember:* with rectal bleeding in middle-aged and older individuals, even in the presence of hemorrhoids, CA *must be ruled out*

What tests help rule out metastases?

CXR, LFTs, others based on history and physical

What are the means by which the CA spreads?

Direct extension: Circumferentially and then through bowel wall to later invade other abdominoperineal organs
Hematogenous: Portal circulation to liver; lumbar/vertebral veins to lungs
Lymphogenous: Regionally
Transperitoneal
Intraluminal

What about CEA?

Carcinoembryonic antigen is *NOT* useful for screening but is useful for baseline and recurrence surveillance (but no proven survival benefit)

What are procedures for prevention/early detection?

1. Annual digital rectal exam starting at age 40 (**remember that approximately 10% of tumors are palpable by rectal exam!)
2. Annual test for fecal occult blood starting at age 40
3. Sigmoidoscopy at ages 50 & 51, then every 3–5 years thereafter.
4. For patients with a family history of familial polyposis, more aggressive monitoring is needed.

How are tumors classified?

Dukes staging: simplified

A: Limited to **mucosa**/submucosa
B: Into the **muscularis propria** or through entire bowel wall
C: (+) Regional **lymph nodes**
D: *D*istant metastasis

Dukes vs. prognosis?	Survival at 5 years
A?	A: ≈80%
B?	B: ≈60%
C?	C: ≈30%
D?	D: ≈5%

What are treatment options? — *Resection:* Wide surgical resection of lesion and its **regional lymphatic drainage;** approach and extent of resection depend on site, extent of tumor

Importance of adjuvant therapy? — It is currently considered standard of care to offer in addition to resection a 5-fluorouracil (5-FU)-based chemotherapy regimen for colon CA and rectal CA if Duke's stage C; in addition, external beam radiation is added to chemo for rectal CA; research has revealed these regimens offer improved local control and increased survival

Postop follow-up? — To most efficiently detect recurrence, the patient should be seen for history, CEA, and physical every 3 months for 2 years, then every 6 months for 2 years. A patient without recurrence at 5 years is most likely clear of disease. However, it is necessary to maintain surveillance of the remainder of the patient's colon as he/she is at risk for other primary tumors. This is accomplished with a screening colonoscopy every 3 years.

What tumor was the Dukes classification originally described for? — Rectal CA

What is the most common cause of colonic obstruction in the adult population? — **Colon cancer!**

DIVERTICULAR DISEASE OF THE COLON

DIVERTICULOSIS

What is diverticulosis? — A condition in which diverticula can be found within the colon; especially the sigmoid colon; the diverticula are actually **false diverticula** in that only mucosa and submucosa herniate through the bowel musculature; true diverticula involve all layers of the bowel wall and are rare in the colon

Describe the pathophysiology	**Weakness** in the bowel wall develops at points where nutrient **blood vessels** enter between antimesenteric and mesenteric taenia; increased intraluminal pressures then cause herniation through these areas
What is the incidence?	Approximately 50–60% in U.S. by age 60, with only 10–20% becoming symptomatic; 95% of people with diverticulosis have **sigmoid** colon involvement
Who is at risk?	People with **low-fiber diets,** chronic constipation, and a positive family history
What are the symptoms/ complications?	*Bleeding*—may be massive *Diverticulitis*—see below *Asymptomatic*—80%; these cases are usually diagnosed incidentally on endoscopy
What is the diagnostic approach?	***Bleeding*** with*OUT* signs of inflammation (fever, increased WBC): must rule out colon CA, therefore endoscopy ***Diverticulitis***—accompanying spasm and infection and/or inflammation; barium enema and endoscopy should be avoided; usually diagnosed by history, but abdominal and/or pelvic CT may be helpful, especially since it may reveal an abscess; barium enema may be done after the inflammation resolves
What is the treatment for diverticulosis?	*Asymptomatic*—high-fiber diet is recommended
Indications for operation with diverticulosis?	Complications of diverticulitis (abscess, fistula, obstruction, stricture, etc.), recurrent episodes, hemorrhage, suspected carcinoma, prolonged symptoms

DIVERTICULITIS

What is it?	Infection or perforation of a diverticulum leading to infection/inflammation of peridiverticular tissue, abscess formation, or generalized peritonitis
Signs/Sx?	LLQ pain (cramping or steady), change in bowel habits (**diarrhea**), fever, chills, anorexia, LLQ mass, nausea, vomiting, and dysuria

What is the key lab finding?	Increased WBC
Radiographic findings?	On x-ray: ileus, partially obstructed colon, air fluid levels, free air if perfed On abdominal/pelvic CT: swollen, edematous bowel wall; this test is particularly helpful to show an abscess that may be a complicating factor
What are barium enema findings?	Barium enema should be avoided in acute setting
What are colonoscopic findings?	Also *should be avoided* in acute cases; colonic spasm increases risk of perforation; this and barium enema may be done after attack subsides
What are complications?	Abscess, peritonitis, fistula (e.g., colovesicular), obstruction
What is initial therapy?	IV fluids, NPO, broad-spectrum antibiotics with anaerobic coverage, NG suction optional
When is surgery warranted?	Abscess, obstruction, fistula, free perforation, sepsis
What surgery is usually done for recurrent bouts of diverticulitis electively?	**A one-stage operation;** resection of the involved segment and primary anastomosis
What surgery is usually performed for an acute case of diverticulitis with a complication of the disease (e.g., abscess, obstruction)?	**A two-staged operation;** resection of the involved segment with an end colostomy and subsequent reanastomosis of the colon
What about mortality?	Operative mortality on admission approximately 5%
How common is massive lower GI bleed with diverticulitis?	Very, very *RARE!* Massive lower GI bleeding is seen with divertic**ulosis!** not diverticulitis!
What is the most common cause of massive lower GI bleeding in the adult population?	Divertic**ulosis** (especially right-sided)

INFLAMMATORY BOWEL DISEASE: CROHN'S DISEASE AND ULCERATIVE COLITIS

Incidence?	High in the Jewish population, low in the black population
Initial symptoms? (4)	Bleeding per rectum (greater in U.C. than in Crohn's), abdominal pain, fever, diarrhea
Extraintestinal manifestations? (7)	Seen in both: (oral) aphthous ulcers, iritis, pyoderma gangrenosum, erythema nodosum, clubbing of fingers, sclerosing cholangitis, arthritis
Anatomical distribution? U.C.	Colon alone (can have "backwash ileitis")
Crohn's	Small bowel alone ≈25%; small bowel and colon ≈ 50%; colon alone ≈ 25%; anal involvement is much more specific for Crohn's; classically said to involve "**mouth to anus**"

Spread?

U.C.	Usually **involves rectum and spreads proximally** in a continuous route *without "skip areas"*
Crohn's	Small bowel and/or colon *with "skip areas,"* and with anal involvement; hence the name "regional enteritis"

Bowel Wall Involvement?

U.C.	Usually confined to **mucosa and submucosa**
Crohn's	****Full thickness** (transmural involvement)

Mucosal Findings?

U.C. (5)	Granular, flat mucosa; ulcers; **crypt abscess;** dilated mucosal vessels; **pseudopolyps**
Crohn's (6)	Aphthoid ulcers; granulomas; linear ulcers; transverse fissures; swollen mucosa; full-thickness wall involvement
Which one has "cobblestoning" on endoscopic exam?	**Crohn's disease**

| Which one has a "lead pipe" appearance on barium enema? | Ulcerative colitis |

Complications? _____

| U.C. | Colonic perforation; **toxic megacolon;** hemorrhage; strictures, obstruction; complications of surgery; and **CANCER** |
| Crohn's | **Anal** fistula; enterocolic fistula; stricture; perforation; abscesses; toxic megacolon; colovesical fistula; enterovaginal fistula; hemorrhage; obstruction |

Cancer Risk? _____

| U.C. | **Approximately 2% per year after the first 10 years of the disease** |
| Crohn's | High risk in areas surgically bypassed from the fecal stream; but also an overall higher risk |

Indications for Surgery? _____

U.C.	**Toxic megacolon;** stricture; CA; *CA prophylaxis;* refractory to medical therapy; increased bleeding; failure of child to mature due to disease and steroids
Crohn's	Refractory to medical therapy; CA; obstruction; massive bleeding; fistula; perforation
What is the medical treatment for IBD?	Sulfa drugs (like **sulfasalazine**) are first-line agents; **steroids** (prednisone) are second-line; these are taken orally unless the patient has rectal involvement alone, for which enemas or suppositories of these agents are helpful; **Flagyl** is being used often for flare-ups

POLYPS

POLYPS OF THE COLON AND RECTUM _____

| What are they? | Tissue growth into the bowel lumen usually consisting of mucosa and/or submucosa |
| How are they anatomically classified? | *Sessile* (flat) = villous
Pedunculated (long-stalked) = adenomatous |

Histologic Classification? _____

Inflammatory (pseudopolyp)?	As in Crohn's or ulcerative colitis
Hamartomatous?	Normal tissue in abnormal configuration; most common is juvenile polyp, which has no malignant potential
Hyperplastic?	Benign with no malignant potential, but significant because of occurrence in areas of neoplastic polyps; must rule out neoplasm
***Neoplastic* (adenomatous)?**	See below; important because they are premalignant or malignant lesions
What determines malignant potential of an adenomatous polyp?	*Size* *Histologic* type *Atypia* of cells
What about size vs. malignancy?	Cancer found in 1 cm adenoma ≈ 1% 1–2 cm adenoma ≈ 10% >2 cm adenoma ≈ 45%
What about histology and cancer potential of an adenomatous polyp?	Tubular ≈5% chance of cancer Tubulovillous ≈20% chance of cancer Villous ≈40% chance of cancer
Which type is most common?	**Adenomatous, approximately 5% of adult population
Where are most polyps found?	**Rectosigmoid colon
What are signs/Sx?	Bleeding (red or dark blood), change in bowel habits, mucus and blood seen in villous types
Diagnostic tests?	Fecal occult blood, CBC, barium enema, endoscope, *Biopsy* of all suspect tissue
Treatment plan?	Endoscopic resection with histologic examination is the first step

POLYPOSIS SYNDROMES _____

What characterizes *familial adenomatous polyposis?*	Hundreds of adenomatous polyps within rectum and colon that begin developing at puberty; all undiagnosed, untreated patients develop CA by age 40–50
Inheritance?	Autosomal dominant

Treatment?	For patients who have only a few adenomas in the rectum, total abdominal colectomy with ileorectal anastomosis is appropriate; these patients will need fairly frequent follow-up for removal of any polyps in the rectum that subsequently develop; for patients who have polyps carpeting the rectum, proctectomy with ileoanal pouch construction
What characterizes *Gardner's syndrome?*	Neoplastic polyps of **small bowel** & colon; CA by age 40 in 100% of undiagnosed patients as in FAP
Treatment?	Same as with FAP
Other associated findings?	**Desmoid** tumors (in the abdominal wall), **osteomas** of skull (seen on x-ray), sebaceous cysts, lipoma, fibroma retroperitoneal fibrosis
What are *juvenile polyps?*	Benign hamartomas in small bowel and colon; not premalignant
What is the significance of *familial juvenile polyposis?*	Benign hamartomas, *but* risk for all GI CAs is increased for the patient and family
What characterizes *Peutz-Jeghers syndrome?*	Hamartomas throughout GI tract; very little malignant potential, but CA risk is increased in other areas
Inheritance?	Autosomal dominant
Other signs?	Melanotic pigmentation of buccal mucosa, lips, digits
Treatment?	Removal of polyps if symptomatic (i.e., bleeding or obstruction)
What is *Cronkite-Canada syndrome?*	Diffuse GI polyps associated with malabsorption/wgt loss and **loss of electrolytes/protein;** signs include **alopecia,** nail atrophy, skin pigmentation
Rx?	Resect for complications
What is Turcot's syndrome?	Colon polyps with malignant CNS tumors (glioblastoma multiforme)

VOLVULUS

What is it?	**Twisting of GI tract** about its mesentery, resulting in obstruction and, if complete, vascular compromise with potential for necrosis and/or perforation

SIGMOID VOLVULUS

Incidence?	Approximately $>\frac{3}{4}$ of colonic volvulus
Etiologic factors?	High-residue diet resulting in bulky stools and tortuous, elongated colon; chronic constipation; laxative abuse; pregnancy; seen most commonly in elderly/bedridden or institutionalized patients; many have Hx of prior abdominal surgery
Signs/Sx?	Progressive abdominal **distention,** anorexia, obstipation; crampy, lower abdominal pain may or may not be present
Abdominal plain film?	Distended loop of bowel, often in the classic "coffee-bean" configuration with convexity pointing to the right
Diagnosis?	Sigmoidoscopy (or radiographic exam with barium)
Barium enema?	Yes, if sigmoidoscopy and plain films fail to confirm the diagnosis; "**bird's beak**" is pathognomonic
Signs of strangulation?	Discolored or hemorrhagic mucosa on sigmoidoscopy, bloody fluid in the rectum, frank ulceration or necrosis at the point of the twist; PERITONEAL signs, fever, hypovolemia, ↑ wbc
Treatment?	If no strangulation, sigmoidoscopic reduction successful in approximately 80% (i.e., **80%** are treated **nonoperatively**); if unsuccessful, barium enema will occasionally reduce; in either case a colonic tube is inserted to serve as a stint and prevent recurrence; without intervention, sigmoid volvulus has a 50% chance of recurrence and many undergo subsequent elective sigmoid resection
What are the indications for surgery?	If strangulation is suspected, or nonoperative reduction unsuccessful, then laparotomy with formation of a colostomy after resection; surgery is also indicated for recurrences, with elective resection of the redundant sigmoid

CECAL VOLVULUS _____

Incidence?	Approximately ¼ of colonic volvulus
Etiology?	Idiopathic poor fixation of the right colon; seen most often in young, healthy adults, many have Hx of abdominal surgery
Signs/Sx?	Colicky pain beginning in the RLQ progressing to a constant pain, vomiting, obstipation, abdominal distention, and small bowel obstruction; many patients will have had previous similar episodes
Diagnosis?	Abdominal plain film; dilated, ovoid colon with large air/fluid level in RLQ, epigastrium, or LUQ (must rule out gastric dilation with NG aspiration)
Barium study?	Not usually necessary and will delay treatment
Treatment?	Uncommonly reducible by colonoscopy; therefore, treated with emergent surgery; if the cecum is viable, cecopexy is performed; if the cecum has infarcted or perforated, right colectomy with primary reanastomosis is performed if feasible (ileostomy may be necessary)
What are the major differences in the management of cecal volvulus vs. sigmoid?	**80% of cecal** volvulus patients require **surgical reduction,** (and almost all (100%) have surgery at some point); **the vast majority of patients with sigmoid volvulus undergo endoscopic reduction of the twist!**

LOWER GI BLEEDING

Definition of LGI bleeding?	Bleeding distal to the ligament of Treitz
Symptoms? (possible)	Abdominal pain, melena, hematochezia, anorexia, fatigue, syncope, SOB
Signs?	BRBPR, Hemoccult +, peritoneal signs, shock, orthostasis, abdominal distention (from obstruction)
Causes?	Diverticular disease (usually **right**-sided in severe hemorrhage), angiodysplasia, colon CA, hemorrhoids, trauma, hereditary hemorrhagic telangiectasia, intussusception,

volvulus, ischemic colitis, IBD (especially ulcerative colitis), anticoagulation, rectal CA, Meckel's diverticulum (with ectopic gastric mucosa), colonic ulcer, chemotherapy, irradiation injury, infarcted bowel, strangulated hernia

Most common cause of massive lower GI bleeding?

****Diverticulosis** (right-sided), # 2 angiodysplasia

Diagnostic tests?

Hx, PE, NG tube aspirate (r/o UGI bleeding must see bile or blood, if not do EGD) then do proctosigmoidoscopy/colonoscopy; proctoscopic exam in E.R.

Must rule out what in patients with lower GI bleeding?

Upper GI bleeding! REMEMBER, NGT ASPIRATION IS NOT 100% (EVEN IF YOU GET BILE WITHOUT BLOOD!) **If any question → EGD**

Lab tests?

CBC, Chem-7, PT/PTT, **type & cross**

Initial treatment?

IVFs: LR, PRBC as needed (through at least 16G peripheral IVs × 2), Foley to follow urine output

Tests to localize bleeding if there is too much blood to see source with scope?

1. Radiolabeled RBC scan—more sensitive for blood loss at rate of 0.1 ml/min
2. Arteriography: need to be bleeding at a rate of >0.5 ml/min

Treatment during angiography?

Infusion of vasopressin—50% successful in nonmassive bleeding; alternative: embolization (rare)

How do you prevent an MI while patient is on vasopressin?

Infusion of nitroglycerin

Treatment if infusion fails?

If bleeding site is known and continues to bleed—elective hemicolectomy

Percentage that spontaneously stop bleeding?

75% stop bleeding with resuscitative measures only

Mortality of initial LGI bleeding?

About 10%

HEMORRHOIDS

What are they?

Engorgement of the venous plexi of the rectum and/or anus, with protrusion of mucosa and/or of the anal margin

Signs/Sx?

Anal mass/prolapse, bleeding, itching, pain

Which type, internal or external, is painful?

External, below dentate line has pain nerve fibers

If a patient has excruciating anal pain and history of hemorrhoids what do they have?

Thrombosed external hemorrhoid!

Causes of hemorrhoids?

Constipation/straining, portal hypertension, pregnancy

CLASSIFICATION BY DEGREES

First degree hemorrhoid?

Hemorrhoids that do not prolapse

Second degree?

Prolapse with defecation but return on their own

Third degree?

Prolapse with defecation or any type of Valsalva maneuver and require active manual reduction (eat fiber!)

Fourth degree?

Prolapsed hemorrhoids that cannot be reduced

Treatment?

High-fiber diet, anal hygiene, topical steroids, sitz baths → rubber band ligation of most (need no anesthetic for internal hemorrhoids) → and surgical resection for large refractory roids

PERIANAL/PERIRECTAL ABSCESS

What is it?

Abscess formation around the anus/rectum

Signs/Sx?

Rectal pain, drainage of pus, fever, perianal mass

Cause?

Crypt abscess in dentate line with spread

Rx?

As with all abscesses (except liver amebic abscesses), **drainage** and +/− antibiotics against colonic flora (especially anaerobes)

27
Liver

What are the divisions of the lobes of the liver and its boundaries?

A line drawn between the gallbladder to just left of the inferior vena cava transects the liver into right and left lobes (Cantlie's line)

What is the hepatic arterial supply?

From the common hepatic artery off the celiac trunk

What is the venous *supply?*

Portal vein (formed from the splenic vein and the superior mesenteric vein)

What is the hepatic venous *drainage?*

Via the hepatic veins, which drain into the IVC

Define the Pringle maneuver?

Compression of the hepatoduodenal ligament and its contents (i.e., hepatic artery and portal vein) to control bleeding from the liver, usually from trauma

What is the maximum amount of liver that can be resected while retaining adequate liver function?

Resection of >80% is compatible with life. If given adequate recovery time, the original mass can be regenerated.

Signs/Sx of liver disease?

Hepatomegaly, splenomegaly, icterus, pruritis (from bile salts in skin), blanching spider telangectasia, gynecomastia, testicular atrophy, caput medusae, dark urine, clay-colored stools, bradycardia, edema, ascites, fever, fetor hepaticus (sweet musty smell), hemorrhoids, variceal bleeding, anemia, body hair loss, liver tenderness

TUMORS OF THE LIVER

What is the most common liver tumor?

Metastatic disease outnumbers primary tumors 20:1. Primary site is usually GI tract.

Labs for work-up of metastatic disease?

LFTs (SGOT and alk phos most useful), CEA for suspected primary colon CA

Imaging studies?

US/CT

What are four types of primary benign liver tumors?	Hemangioma (most common) Hepatocellular **ADENOMA**—strongly associated with birth control pills and anabolic steroids Focal nodular hyperplasia Infantile hemangioendothelioma
What are four types of primary malignant liver tumors?	Hepatocellular **CARCINOMA** Hepatoblastoma (in children!) Cholangiocarcinoma (CA of the bile duct epithelium) Angiosarcoma—(associated with vinyl chloride exposure)

HEPATOCELLULAR ADENOMA

What is it?	Benign liver tumor
Histology?	Hepatocytes
Risk factors?	Women, **birth control pills**
Sx/Signs?	RUQ pain/mass, shock
Complications?	Rupture with bleeding, necrosis
Dx?	CT, U/S
Rx?	Stop birth control pills→may shrink, resect if symptomatic or if large because of increased chance of hemorrhage/necrosis

FOCAL NODULAR HYPERPLASIA

What is it?	Benign liver tumor similar to hepatocellular adenoma
Risk factors?	Women
Associated with birth control pills?	No
Dx?	U/S, CT
Rx?	Resect if symptomatic

HEPATIC HEMANGIOMA

What is it?	Benign vascular tumor of liver
Claim to infamy?	**Most common benign liver tumor!**
Sx/signs?	RUQ pain/mass, shock, CHF

Complications?	Hemorrhage, congestive heart failure, coagulopathy
Dx?	CT with IV contrast
Biopsy?	Do not—chance of severe hemorrhage with biopsy
Rx?	Resect if symptomatic

Hepatocellular Carcinoma _____

Incidence?	Most common primary malignant liver tumor (>$\frac{3}{4}$ of all primary malignant tumors)
Population at risk?	Highest rate in Africa and Asia
Associated risk factors?	**Cirrhosis,** hepatitis B virus, ETOH abuse, hemochromatosis, schistosomiasis, aflatoxin (fungi), α-1-antitrypsin deficiency
Sx/Signs?	Dull RUQ pain, hepatomegaly, abd mass, weight loss, paraneoplastic syndromes
Labs?	Elevated α-fetoprotein
Most common site of metastasis?	Lungs
Rx and prognosis?	**Poor!** surgically resectable; about 1 in 10 live 5 years (clinical trials with transplantation)
Which liver enzymes are made by hepatocytes?	AST and ALT
What is the source of alkaline phosphatase?	**Ductal epithelium**
Subtype that has a better prognosis?	Fibrolamellar hepatoma (young adults)

LIVER ABSCESSES

Etiology?	1. Direct spread from gall bladder/biliary tract 2. Portal spread from GI infection (e.g., appendicitis, diverticulitis) 3. Systemic source (bacteremia) 4. Cryptogenic
What are the two most common types?	Bacterial (most common in U.S.) and amoebic (most common worldwide)

Define pyogenic?	Caused by bacteria
Define cryptogenic?	Unknown/puzzling (cryptic)
DDx of liver abscess?	Pyogenic (bacterial), parasitic, fungal

BACTERIAL

What are the three most common organisms?	*E. coli, Bacteroides,* anaerobic streptococci, mixed
Signs/Sx?	Sepsis, **fever, chills,** leukocytosis, **RUQ pain,** increased LFTs
Rx?	IV antibiotics/percutaneous drainage/surgical drainage if multiple/loculated or failed multiple percutaneous attempts

AMOEBIC

Etiology?	*Entamoeba histolytica,* typically reaches liver via portal vein from intestinal amebiasis
Risk factors?	Patient from country below the U.S. border with Mexico, institutions
Signs/Sx?	Same as bacterial with most involving the R lobe of the liver (''**anchovy paste pus**'' present in the abscess)
Labs?	Indirect hemagglutination titers for *Entamoeba* antibodies elevated in >95%
Rx?	**Metronidazole IV,** surgical drainage is **controversial**

Hydatid Liver Cysts

What is it?	Usually a right lobe cyst filled with *Echinococcus (Echinococcus granulosus,* think granule = cyst), parasite
Risks?	Travel, exposure to dogs
Dx?	Indirect hemagglutination antibody test
Findings on AXR?	Calcified outline of cyst
What is the risk of surgical removal of echinococcal (hydatid) cysts?	Rupture or leakage of cyst contents into the abdomen may cause a fatal **anaphylactic** reaction.

Rx?

Surgical resection; large cysts can be drained after injection of toxic substance into the cyst (hypertonic saline)

PORTAL HYPERTENSION

Pathophysiology?

Elevated portal pressure (nl pressure is about 6 mm Hg) caused by distortion of normal parenchyma by regenerating hepatic nodules

What is the most common physical finding in patients with cirrhosis?

Splenomegaly

Associated clinical findings in portal HTN?

Caput medusa, hemorrhoids, splenomegaly, esophageal varices

How is portal pressure measured?

Indirect hepatic vein wedge pressure (analogous to PCWP), or in O.R. Directly

What constitutes the portal-systemic collateral circulation in portal hypertension? (4)

1. Coronary veins draining into the azygous system (esophageal varices—develop when pressure >20 mm Hg) = **esophageal varices**
2. Umbilical vein draining into the epigastric veins = **caput medusae**
3. Small mesenteric veins (veins of Retzius) draining retroperitoneally into lumbar veins
4. Superior hemorrhoidal vein (which normally drains into the inferior mesenteric vein) draining into the middle and inferior hemorrhoidal veins (causing internal hemorrhoids) = **hemorrhoids**

Etiology?

Cirrhosis (85%), schistosomiasis, hepatitis, Budd-Chiari syndrome, hemochromatosis, Wilson's disease (elevated copper)

What is Budd-Chiari syndrome?

Thrombosis of the hepatic veins (major cause of UGI bleeding in children!)

What percentage of alcoholics develop cirrhosis?

Surprising, <1 in 5

What percentage of cirrhotics develop esophageal varices?

Slightly more than ⅓

How many cirrhotics with esophageal varices have documented bleeding?

About ⅓

In cirrhotics with known varices and suffering upper GI bleeding, how often is that bleeding due to the varices?

Only about ½! the vast majority of the other causes include Gastritis, peptic ulcer disease, and Mallory-Weiss

Workup and Rx for variceal bleeding?

1. As with all upper GI bleeding: IV fluid, Foley, NG tube/H_2O lavage
2. EGD SCOPE—(remember bleeding due to varices only ½ the time)
3. If varices with active bleeding, then IV vasopressin (and nitroglycerin to avoid MI)
4. Balloon tamponade (Blakemore-Sengstaken balloon)
5. EGD with sclerotherapy
6. Refractory bleeding after repeated sclerotherapy/balloon tamponade = portacaval shunt or liver transplantation

Surgical Shunts?

Selective Shunt
   Distal Splenorenal (Warren shunt): #1 elective shunt procedure; lowest incidence of encephalopathy postop because only the splenic flow is diverted to decompress the varices
Nonselective shunts
   1. **End-to-side shunt:** Portal vein to IVC
   2. **Mesocaval shunt:** Graft from SMV to IVC
   3. **Side-to-side shunt:** Side of portal vein anastomosed to IVC—partially preserves portal flow
   4. Synthetic H-graft (easier to transplant patient later)
   5. *TIPS:* transjugular intrahepatic portal caval shunt (angiographic procedure)

What is the Warren shunt?

Distal splenorenal shunt—(must also tie off coronary vein)

Most common perioperative cause of death following shunt procedure?

Hepatic failure secondary to decreased blood flow (accounts for ⅔ of deaths); also increases incidence of hepatic encephalopathy

What is Child's class?

A classification system that estimates hepatic reserve in patients with hepatic failure

What comprises the Child's classification?

Lab: bilirubin, albumin
Clinical: nutrition, encephalopathy, ascites

Define Child's classification	Bili	ALB	Nutrit	Enceph	Ascites
A?	<2	>3.5	excellent	none	none
B?	2–3	3.–3.5	good	minimal	easily cont
C?	>3	<3	poor	severe	poorly cont

Think, as in a letter grading system, A is better than B, B is better than C

Operative mortality for venocaval shunt by Child's classification

A?   <5% mortality

B?   <15%

C?   about ⅓ die

What is hemobilia?   Blood draining via common bile duct

Sx/signs of hemobilia?   Triad: 1. RUQ pain
                                   2. Guaiac +/upper GI bleeding
                                   3. Jaundice

Causes?   Trauma, PTC, tumors, etc.

What vitamin should every liver failure patient with a coagulopathy receive?   Vitamin K! (Remember: 2, 7, 9, 10 are liver clotting factors)

Radiographic evaluations?	**Abdominal films:** about 10% of all stones, 50% of pigmented stones are radiopaque; may see air in biliary tree in cases of fistula formation (for comparison, approx. 80% of kidney stones and about 5% of patients with appendicitis will have radiopaque fecaliths)
	Ultrasound: may show stones, sludge, thickened walls, etc
	Endoscopic retrograde cholangiopancreatography (ERCP): allows radiographic visualization and biopsy of ducts/brush for cytology/papillotomy via duodenum
	Percutaneous transhepatic cholangiography (PTC): contrast study
	HIDA/PRIDA scan: radioisotope evaluation can show cystic duct obstruction
Initial diagnostic study of choice for evaluation of the biliary tract/cholelithiasis?	**ULTRASOUND!**

CHOLELITHIASIS

What is it?	The formation of gallstones
Risk factors?	"Five F's"—female, fat, forty, fertile (multiparity), flatulent (malabsorption of fat leads to gas production by intestinal flora); also oral contraceptives, bile stasis, chronic hemolysis (pigment stones), cirrhosis, infection, native American heritage, rapid wgt loss, obesity, IBD, ileal resection, TPN, duodenal diverticulum, vagotomy, ↑age
Two types of stones?	1. Cholesterol stones (75% of all stones) 2. Pigment stones (25% of all stones)
Pathogenesis of cholesterol stones?	Secretion of bile supersaturated with cholesterol

Rx?	**Cholecystectomy if symptomatic
What is choledocholithiasis?	**Gallstones in the bile ducts**
Which artery is susceptible to injury during cholecystectomy?	R. hepatic artery, secondary to its proximity to the cystic artery
What is the name of the valves of the gallbladder?	Spiral valves of Heister
Where is the infundibulum of the gallbladder?	Near the cystic duct
Where is the fundus of the gallbladder?	The end of the gallbladder
Define the triangle of CALOT	Bounded by 1. Cystic duct 2. Common hepatic duct 3. Inferior border of the liver
What is found in the triangle of CALOT?	**Cystic artery** and the right hepatic artery

ACUTE CHOLECYSTITIS

Pathogenesis?	Obstruction of cystic duct leads to inflammation of the gallbladder; about 95% due to calculi and about 5% due to acalculus obstruction
Risks?	Same as for formation of gallstones
Sx/signs?	RUQ pain/tenderness, fatty food intolerance (recurrence of Sx) due to cholecystokinin stimulation of the obstructed gallbladder, fever, N/V, *painful* palpable gallbladder in 33%, icterus uncommon, positive Murphy's sign, right subscapular pain (referred), epigastric discomfort (referred)
What is Murphy's sign?	Acute pain and inspiratory arrest elicited by **palpation of the RUQ** during inspiration
Complications?	Abscess, perforation, choledocholithiasis, cholecystenteric fistula formation
Labs?	Increased WBC, bilirubin, amylase, and alk phos (all not always elevated)
Dx tests?	**U/S

Rx?   IVFs, abx, NG tube decompression, **Cholecystectomy,** or if poor operative candidate: cholecystostomy

ACUTE ACALCULUS CHOLECYSTITIS

What is it?   Acute cholecystitis without evidence of stones

Pathogenesis?   Believed to be due to sludge and gallbladder disuse, perhaps secondary to absence of cholecystokinin stimulation (decreased contraction of gallbladder)

Risk factors?   Prolonged fasting, TPN, often occurs in prolonged postop or ICU setting (e.g., trauma, multiple transfusions)

Dx test?   U/S—sludge and inflammation present

Mortality?   90% if undiagnosed

CHOLANGITIS

What is it?   Bacterial infection of the biliary tract due to obstruction (either partial or complete); potentially life-threatening

Common causes of Obx?   *Choledocholithiasis*, stricture (usually postop), neoplasm (usually ampullary carcinoma), or extrinsic compression (pancreatic pseudocyst)

Signs/Sx?   Charcot's triad—fever/chills, RUQ pain, and jaundice
Reynold's pentad—Charcot's plus altered mental status and shock

Labs?   Increased WBC, bili, and alk phos; ±blood cx **amylase is normal

Common organisms?   *E. coli* **most common;** others include *Klebsiella, Pseudomonas,* enterococci, *Proteus,* and in approx. ¼ cases anaerobes: *B. fragilis* (#1), *C. perfringens*

Dx tests?   **Ultrasound immediately, followed by a contrast study (i.e., PTC or ERCP) after patient has "cooled off" with IV antibiotics**

| What is suppurative cholangitis? | Severe infection with sepsis "pus under pressure" |
| Rx? | **Nonsuppurative: antibiotics with definitive Rx later**
Suppurative: antibiotics/decompression pronto; decompression can be obtained by either ERCP with papillotomy, PTC with catheter drainage, or laparotomy with T-tube placement |

SCLEROSING CHOLANGITIS

What is it?	Fibrous thickening of bile duct walls creates "**beads on a string**" appearance on contrast study; progressive obstruction leads to cirrhosis and liver failure
Etiology?	Unknown, but 40% associated with inflammatory bowel disease
Rx?	1. Hepatoenteric anastomosis (if primarily extrahepatic ducts involved) 2. Transplant (if primarily intrahepatic disease or advanced cirrhosis)

GALLSTONE ILEUS

What is it?	SBO due to a large (> 2.5 cm) gallstone that has eroded through the gallbladder and into the duodenum/small bowel; i.e., a gallstone creates a cholecystenteric fistula and lodges in the ileocecal valve, causing obstruction
Population at risk?	Most commonly seen in **women over 70 y.o.**
Signs/Sx?	Sx of SBO—distention, vomiting, hypovolemia, RUQ pain, and (rarely) a palpable stone
DDx?	Other causes of SBO, cholangitis, mesenteric ischemia, appendicitis (always in the differential unless it has been removed!)
Diagnostic test?	*Abd x-ray:* occasionally see radiopaque gallstone in the bowel, ****40% have air in the biliary tract**, SB distention and air fluid levels secondary to ileus *UGI:* used if Dx in question and will show cholecystenteric fistula and the obstruction

Rx?	Surgery—enterotomy with removal of the stone and cholecystectomy/closure of fistula

CARCINOMA OF THE GALLBLADDER

What is it?	Malignant neoplasm arising in the gallbladder: very low incidence ¾ are **adenocarcinoma** Rest are undifferentiated, squamous cell, mixed carcinomas
Risks?	*Gallstones* (present or by history in approx. 100% of cases), cholecystenteric fistula, **porcelain gallbladder**, adenomas, ulcerative colitis, native American heritage, and advancing age
Sx?	Similar to benign biliary tract disease, plus pain, weight loss, anorexia
Signs?	Jaundice (from invasion of the common duct or compression by involved pericholedochal lymph nodes), RUQ mass, palpable gallbladder (advanced disease)
Dx?	Abdominal CT, ERCP
Complications?	Metastases, perforation of the GB, fistulization, GI/biliary tract obstruction, GI hemorrhage
Prognosis?	**Very poor** —>¾ die within 1 year of diagnosis, primarily because disease is discovered late —5% five-year survival (most of these are discovered incidently at cholecystectomy for benign disease)
Rx?	Resect if possible, relieve obstructions with resections/bypass
What is Courvoisier's GB?	A palpable, *nontender* (unlike acute cholecystitis) **gallbladder** associated with cancer of the head of the pancreas, able to distend because it has not been scarred down by gallstones

CHOLANGIOCARCINOMA

What is it?	Malignancy of the extrahepatic or intrahepatic ducts, primarily adenocarcinoma

Sx? signs?

Usually as biliary obstruction, jaundice, etc.

What is a Klatskin tumor?

Tumor that involves the junction of the right and left hepatic ducts; commonly presents with Sx of gradual obstruction

What is a porcelain gallbladder?

Calcified gallbladder seen on AXR; due to chronic cholelithiasis/cholecystitis with calcified scar tissue in gallbladder wall; **cholecystectomy** is required due to the strong association of **gallbladder carcinoma** with this condition

What is hydrops of the gallbladder?

Complete obstruction of the cystic duct by a gallstone, with filling of the gallbladder with fluid (not bile) from the gallbladder mucosa

Air in the biliary tract and SBO in a women >70 years of age is what until proven otherwise?

Gallstone ileus

29
Pancreas

Regions of the pancreas? Head, uncinate process, neck (in front of the SMV), body, tail

Name the pancreatic ducts Wirsung
Santorini

Which duct is the main duct? Duct of Wirsung is the major duct (Think: *S*antorini = *S*mall)

Blood supply to head of the pancreas?
1. Celiac→gastroduodenal→I. anterior superior pancreaticoduodenal artery, II. posterior superior pancreaticoduodenal artery
2. Superior mesenteric artery→I. anterior inferior pancreaticoduodenal artery, II. posterior inferior pancreaticoduodenal artery

Why must you remove the duodenum if you remove the head of the pancreas? They share the same blood supply

Endocrine function of the pancreas? Islets of Langerhans
alpha cells: glucagon
beta cells: insulin

Exocrine function of the pancreas? AMYLASE, lipase, trypsin/chymotrypsin, carboxypeptidase

PANCREATITIS

ACUTE PANCREATITIS

What is it? Inflammation of pancreas caused by autodigestion by its own activated enzymes

Risks? **Gallstones, ETOH,** Together account for 85% of all cases
Hypercalcemia
Trauma
Hyperlipidemia
Iatrogenic (ERCP)

143

Cardiopulmonary bypass (decreased blood flow)

Familial

Drugs (thiazide diuretics, steroids)

Scorpion sting (found on an exotic island—favorite on rounds)

Idiopathic

Infectious (coxsackie, mumps)

Symptoms?   Epigastric **pain** (frequently radiates to another quadrant or back); nausea and vomiting

Signs of pancreatitis?   Epigastric tenderness
Epigastric mass
Decreased bowel sounds (adynamic ileus)
Fever
Dehydration/shock

DDx?   Gastritis/PUD
Perforated viscus
Acute cholecystitis
SBO
Mesenteric infarction
Ruptured AAA
Biliary colic
Inferior M.I.

DDx increased amylase?   Salivary tumor
Liver disease
Renal failure
SBO
Ovarian tumor
Ectopic pregnancy
Macroamylasemia

Labs to order?   CBC
LFT
Amylase/lipase
T&C
ABG
Ca^{2+}
Glucose/electrolytes

Diagnostic tests?   H&P—h/o ETOH or gallstones/risk factors
Labs—High amylase, high WBC, high lipase
X-ray—Sentinel loop, colon cutoff, gallstones (only 10% visible on x-ray)
U/S—Pseudocyst, phlegmon, abscess
CT—Pseudocyst, phlegmon, abscess

Treatment?	NPO
	NG tube
	IVF
	TPN
	H2 blocker
	Analgesia (DEMEROL, not morphine—less sphincter of Oddi spasm)
	Eradication of biliary dz/ETOH
Prognosis?	Based on *Ranson's criteria*

Ranson's Criteria

At presentation?	1. Age >55
	2. WBC >16000
	3. Glc >200
	4. AST >250
	5. LDH >350
During initial 48 hr?	1. Base deficit >4
	2. BUN increase >5 mg/dl
	3. Fluid sequestration >6 L
	4. Serum Ca^{2+} <8
	5. Hct decrease >10%
	6. PO_2 (ABG) <60 mm Hg
	Amylase value is *NOT* one of Ranson's criteria!
Mortality per positive criteria?	
0–2	0–2 <5%
3–4	3–4 ≈20%
5–6	5–6 ≈40%
7–8	7–8 ≈100%
Complications?	**Pseudocyst**
	Abscess
	Splenic/mesenteric/portal vessel rupture or thrombosis
	Pancreatic ascites
	ARDS/sepsis
Complication of splenic vein thrombosis?	Gastric varices

Hemorrhagic Pancreatitis

What?	Bleeding into parenchyma and surrounding retroperitoneal structures with extensive pancreatic necrosis
Signs?	*Cullen's*—periumbilical
	Grey Turner's—flank

DEFINE

Cullen's sign	Bluish discoloration of the periumbilical area due to retroperitoneal hemorrhage tracking around to the anterior abdominal wall through fascial planes
Grey Turner's sign	Ecchymosis or discoloration of the flank in patients with retroperitoneal hemorrhage (due to dissecting blood from the retroperitoneum)

CHRONIC PANCREATITIS

What?

Inflammation of pancreas caused by autodigestion by its own activated enzymes causing **destruction** of the parenchyma with **fibrosis** and calcification leading to eventual decrease in endocrine and exocrine function

Risks?

ETOH (#1)—vast majority
Few: Hypercalcemia
      Hyperlipidemia
      Familial
      Trauma
      Iatrogenic
      Gallstones

Symptoms?

Chronic, waxing and waning abd pain with radiation to back; can get acute attacks superimposed on chronic pattern

Signs?

IDDM (up to $\frac{1}{3}$)
Steatorrhea (up to $\frac{1}{4}$)
Ascites
Pleural effusion (usually L-sided)

DDx?

Pancreatic cancer

Labs?

Amylase/lipase
72-hr fecal fat analysis
Glc tolerance test (IDDM)

Diagnostic tests?

H&P—**ETOH**
CT—Has greatest sensitivity for gland enlargement/atrophy, calcifications, masses, pseudocysts
KUB—Calcification in pancreas
ERCP—Ductal irregularities with dilation and stenosis (*Chain of Lakes*), pseudocysts

Treatment?	Medical
	Stop ETOH use!—can stop attacks, though parenchymal damage continues secondary to ductal obstruction and fibrosis
	Insulin for IDDM
	Pancreatic enzyme replacement
	Narcotics for pain (WATCH FOR ADDICTION!)
	Surgical
	Peustow—longitudinal pancreaticojejunostomy
	DuVal—distal pancreaticojejunostomy
Complications?	IDDM
	Steatorrhea
	Malnutrition
	Biliary obstruction
	Splenic vein thrombosis →
	Hypersplenism
	Gastric varices
	Pancreatic pseudocyst/abscess
	Narcotic addiction
	Pancreatic ascites/pleural effusion

PANCREATIC ASCITES/PLEURAL EFFUSION

What is it?	Fluid collections formed by pancreatic duct disruption and subsequent accumulation of pancreatic secretions
Risks?	Occurs with acute or chronic pancreatitis
	Trauma
Diagnostic tests?	Paracentesis/thoracentesis
	Amylase level of fluid
	ERCP to locate disrupted duct, if fluid continues to accumulate
Treatment?	Nonoperative
	Paracentesis
	Thoracentesis or chest tube
	NPO/supportive
	Surgical—If not resolved in 3 weeks
	Distal pancreatectomy
	Roux-en-Y pancreaticojejunostomy

PANCREATIC PSEUDOCYST

What is it?	Encapsulated collection of pancreatic fluid (''pseudo'' = wall formed by inflammatory fibrosis, **NOT epithelial cell lining**)
Incidence?	About 1 in 10 after alcoholic pancreatitis
Risks?	Acute pancreatitis
Symptoms?	**Epigastric pain**** Mild fever Weight loss Suspect when patient with acute pancreatitis fails to resolve pain
Signs?	Palpable epigastric **mass;** tender epigastrium
Labs?	Amylase/lipase Bilirubin CBC
Diagnostic tests?	Labs—High amylase, leukocytosis, high bili (if obstruction) **U/S**—Fluid-filled mass (best study) **CT**—Fluid-filled mass, good for showing multiple cysts **ERCP**—Radiopaque material fills cyst(s)
DDx of a pseudocyst?	Cystadenocarcinoma
Complications of pancreatic pseudocyst?	Infection, bleeding into cyst, fistula
Treatment?	Treat pancreatitis; drain after 6 weeks internally or by percutaneous external route
Wait how long before drainage of pseudocyst?	6 weeks for pseudocyst walls to ''**mature**'' or become firm enough to hold sutures
Prognosis?	Increased recurrence with external drainage

PANCREATIC CARCINOMA

What is it?	Adenocarcinoma of the pancreas arising from duct cells
Risks?	**Age and smoking;** diabetes mellitus, heavy alcohol use, the chemicals benzidine and β-naphthylamine may be associated
Type?	Over 90% are duct cell adenocarcinomas; others include cystadenocarcinoma and acinar cell carcinoma

Location?	⅔ arise in the head of the pancreas; ⅓ in the body and tail

Signs/Sx?	Depend on location of the tumor:
	    Head of pancreas: ***Painless jaundice*** secondary to obstruction of the bile duct, wgt loss and abdominal pain, weakness, pruritis (from jaundice = bile salts), anorexia, palpable nontender gallbladder (**Courvoisier's sign**), acholic stools (clay-colored), and dark urine
	    Tumors arising in the body or tail: present with wgt loss and pain (90%), migratory thrombophlebitis (10%), and jaundice in less than 10% of cases

Labs?	**Increased direct bilirubin and alkaline phos** (as a result of biliary obstruction), ± increased LFTs, and increased CEA in advanced disease; increased amylase **not** frequently seen
Dx studies?	U/S (good screening study), abdominal CT cholangiography (PTC or ERCP with possible bx, selective angiography (for staging and defining arterial and venous involvement and anatomy)
Rx?	Resection if feasible Head of pancreas CA—Whipple Tail/body—distal resection
Prognosis?	**Dismal,** with 90% of patients dying within 1 yr of diagnosis; overall <5% 5-yr survival

MISCELLANEOUS PANCREAS

What is an annular pancreas?	Pancreas encircles the duodenum; bypass if obstruction, do **not resect**
What is pancreatic divisum?	Failure of the two pancreatic ducts to fuse; the normally small duct (**s**mall = **S**antorini) of Santorini acts as the main duct in pancreatic divisum (Think: The 2 pancreatic ducts are *divided* = *divisum*)
What is heterotopic pancreatic tissue?	Heterotopic submucosal pancreatic tissue found in stomach, intestine, duodenum
What is a Peustow?	Longitudinal filleting of the pancreas with a side-to-side anastomosis with the small bowel

30
Breast Cancer

What is it?	Carcinoma of the breast
Incidence?	One in 10 American women develop breast cancer
Risk factors?	Family hx, nulliparity or first pregnancy late; CA in ipsilateral/opposite breast, early menarche, late menopause (to remember **early** menarche and **late** menopause: think of these two as allowing more time for the breast to have to go through the changes of menses)
Symptoms?	Mass, pain (**most painless**), nipple discharge, local edema, nipple retraction, dimple, nipple rash
Why skin retraction?	Tumor involvement of Cooper's ligaments
Signs?	Mass: best time to examine breast is a week after menstrual period; 1 cm is the smallest lesion that can be palpated on examination; ½ of cancers start in upper outer quadrant; dimple, nipple rash, edema, axillary/supraclavicular nodes
Most common site of CA?	**Upper outer quadrants**
Most common type of CA?	**Infiltrating ductal carcinoma**
DDx?	Fibrocystic disease of the breast, fibroadenoma, intraductal papilloma, duct ectasia, fat necrosis, Abscess
Screening?	20–40 breast exam q 2–3 years by a physician; >40 annual breast exam mammographic recommendations are changing; check to see latest recommendations! • All women >20 you are encouraged to self-examine breasts monthly.

Why is mammography more helpful in older women?	Because breast tissue undergoes fatty replacement with age and masses are more easily visible; younger women have more fibrous tissue making mammogram harder to interpret
Diagnostic tests?	• All suspicious masses should be biopsied! • Needle biopsy—15% false-negative rate (negative needle biopsy should **always** be followed by an open biopsy) • Open biopsy—preferred method; small lesions should be completely excised
Indications for biopsy?	Persistent mass after aspiration Solid mass Blood in cyst aspirate Suspicious lesion by mammography Bloody nipple discharge Ulcer or dermatitis of nipple
How to biopsy a nonpalpable mass seen on mammogram?	Needle localization by radiologist, followed by biopsy; removed breast tissue must be checked by mammogram to ensure all of suspicious lesion has been excised
Hormone receptors?	Presence or absence of estrogen and progesterone receptors is key to the management and prognosis of metastatic breast CA
What staging system is used?	TMN: tumor/mets/nodes
Staging?	*Simplified:*
Stage I	<2 cm tumor without metastases, **no nodes**
Stage II	Tumor 2–5 cm in diameter with + mobile nodes, no mets

Stage III	1. Tumor >5 cm
	2. Also any of the following:
	    Peau d'Orange
	    Chest wall invasion/fixation
	    Inflammatory cancer
	    Breast skin ulceration
	    Breast skin satellite mets
	    Fixed axillary nodes

Stage IV	Any size tumor, any # of nodes, with **distant** metastases

What nerves must surgeon beware of (4)?

1. **Long thoracic**—from brachial plexus, courses along lat chest wall in midaxillary line to serratus anterior; damage leads to winging of scapula
2. **Thoracodorsal**—innervation to latissimus dorsi; weakness in adduction, extension, int. rotation of humerus
3. **Med. thoracic**—innervation to pec minor and pec major (A.K.A. med. pectoral n.)
4. **Lat. thoracic**—innervation to pec major (A.K.A. lat. pectoral n.)

Metastases?

75% to ipsilateral **lymph nodes;** bloodborne mets frequently go to bone (upper femur, pelvis, spine, skull, ribs) as well as lung, liver, brain

Levels of axillary lymph nodes?

Level I (low)—lateral to pec minor
Level II (middle)—deep to pec minor
Level III (high)—medial/superior to pec minor
   Higher level of involvement has worse prognosis, but this is not as important as number of positive nodes (think, the levels I, II, III are in the same superior-inferior anatomic order as the Leforte facial fractures and the trauma neck zones—"I dare you to forget!")

What are Rotter's nodes?

Nodes between the pectoralis major and the pectoralis minor muscles; not usually removed unless clinical evidence of mets

What is the most common cause of a bloody nipple discharge in a young woman?

Intraductal papilloma

What are the suspensory breast ligaments called?

Cooper's ligaments

Description of the edema of the dermis in inflammatory carcinoma of the breast?

Peau d'orange (orange peel)

Most common breast tumor in patients under 30 years old?

Fibroadenoma

Most common cause of breast mass after blunt breast trauma?

Fat necrosis

What is DCIS?	Ductal carcinoma in situ, A.K.A. intraductal carcinoma
What is LCIS?	Lobular carcinoma in situ
With LCIS, which breast is at risk for subsequent breast cancer?	**Equal** risk of recurrence in **both** the ipsilateral and contralateral breast!
How does one Rx a breast cyst?	Needle drainage; if bloody→ open bx; if straw/green follow unless it recurs→ bx
Most common cause of green nipple discharge?	Fibrocystic disease
What is a lumpectomy and radiation?	Segmental mastectomy (removal of a part of the breast); **axillary node dissection and course of radiation therapy *after* operation**
What is a modified radical mastectomy?	Removal of the breast, axillary nodes and nipple; pectoralis major and minor are not removed (Auchincloss); drains are placed to drain lymph fluid
What is a simple mastectomy?	Removal of the breast without removal of the axillary nodes
Complications after modified radical mastectomy?	Ipsilateral arm **lymphedema,** infection
How does tamoxifen work?	Binds estrogen receptors
Guidelines for breast exam by a physician?	20–40 years of age: every 3 years Over 40 years: exam every year

Boundaries of the axilla for dissection
    Superior?
    Posterior?
    Lateral?
    Medial?
	
	Axillary vein
	Long thoracic nerve
	Latissimus
	Depends on the level of nodes taken (I, II, III)

Define clinical presentation of a fibroadenoma	Young women <30 years; solid, mobile, **well-circumscribed** round mass; Rx by surgical resection
What is cystosarcoma phyllodes?	A subgroup of Fibroadenoma, that is very aggressive and malignant
What is Paget's disease of the breast?	Scaling rash/dermatitis of the nipple caused by invasion of skin by cells from a ductal carcinoma

31
Endocrine Surgery

NORMAL ADRENAL PHYSIOLOGY

What is ACTH?

Adrenocorticotropic hormone: released normally by the anterior pituitary, which in turn causes release of cortisol by the adrenal

What feeds back to inhibit ACTH secretion?

Cortisol

How does one indirectly measure cortisol levels over a short duration?

By measuring urine cortisol or the breakdown product of cortisol: 17-hydroxycorticosteroid (**17-OHCS**) in the urine

CUSHING'S SYNDROME

What is Cushing's syndrome?

Excessive **cortisol** production

What is Cushing's disease?

Cushing's syndrome caused by excess production of ACTH by the **pituitary**

What is an adrenal source of Cushing's syndrome?

Adrenal tumor that secretes cortisol regardless of ACTH level

What is an ectopic ACTH source?

A tumor not found in the pituitary that secretes ACTH, which in turn causes a release of cortisol by the adrenal

Signs/Sx of Cushing's syndrome?

Truncal obesity, hirsutism, "moon" facies, acne, "buffalo hump," purple striae, HTN, diabetes, weakness, depression, easy bruisability, myopathy

Causes?

Pituitary malfunction, adrenal adenoma, adrenal carcinoma, ectopic ACTH-producing tumor; Thus, primary cortisol secretion or cortisol secretion caused by elevated levels of ACTH

What is the dexamethasone suppression test?

Dexamethasone is a **cortisol analog** that suppresses pituitary secretion of ACTH and thus cortisol in normal individuals

What is the metyrapone stimulation test?	Metyrapone is an **inhibitor of cortisol** production (inhibits 11b-hydroxylase, if you must know); the decrease in cortisol results in an increase in ACTH and, subsequently and finally, an increase in serum cortisol in normals and patients with Cushing's disease
Differentiating lab tests for adrenal source of Cushing's syndrome?	**ACTH undetectable** and FAILURE to suppress urinary 17-OHCS with high-dose dexamethasone suppression test; metyrapone stimulation test reveals no increase in cortisol
Imaging for adrenal source for Cushing's syndrome?	Imaging with CT and iodocholesterol scintigraphy
Differentiating lab tests for Cushing's disease?	**ACTH normal or elevated;** dexamethasone suppression to <50% of ''baseline'' (but ACTH levels will be elevated during some part of the day); metyrapone stim test results in an increase in cortisol
Differentiating lab tests for ectopic ACTH tumor?	**ACTH elevated;** failure to suppress with dexamethasone suppression test and metyrapone stim test reveals no increase in cortisol
Most common site of ectopic ACTH-producing tumor?	More than ⅔ are oat cell tumors of the lung

Treatment _____

Adrenal adenoma?	Unilateral adrenalectomy, since they are almost always UNILATERAL
Adrenal carcinoma?	Surgical excision; only ⅓ of cases are operable
Ectopic ACTH producing tumor?	Surgical excision if feasible
What is mitotane?	Medication that selectively **kills the cells that produce cortisol** (kills zona fasciculata and zona reticularis); used in nonoperative cases of adrenal carcinoma
What is Nelson's syndrome?	Pituitary hypersecretion occurring in ≈20% of all Cushing's patients s/p adrenalectomy leading to hyperpigmentation, headache, exophthalmos, ↑ sex hormones, and pituitary enlargement leading to visual field deficits/blindness; (think of it as an acute loss of the abnormal massive negative cortisol feedback)

ADRENAL INCIDENTALOMA

What is an incidentaloma?

A tumor found in the adrenal cortex **incidentally** on a CT scan done for an unrelated reason

Risk factor for carcinoma?

Solid tumor >6 cm in diameter

Treatment?

Controversial for smaller/medium-sized tumors; but all would agree with surgical resection of solid incidentalomas >6 cm in diameter

PHEOCHROMOCYTOMA

What is it?

Tumor of the adrenal medulla and other similar tissues (e.g., sympathetic ganglion) that produces **catecholamines** (epi, norepi, dopamine)

Incidence?

It is the cause of HTN in ≈1/500 hypertensives (≈10% of the U.S. population has HTN)

Affected age groups? (2)

Any age; children and adults avg age = 40–60.

Signs/Sx?

HYPERTENSION
All are due to increased catechols: "classic" Sx triad: headache, episodic diaphoresis, and palpitations; also, HTN (50%), pallor → flushing, anxiety, weight loss, tachycardia, hyperglycemia

Differential Dx?

Renovascular HTN, menopause, migraine headache, carcinoid syndrome, preeclampsia, neuroblastoma, anxiety disorder with panic attacks, hyperthyroidism, insulinoma

Lab tests?

Urine screen: Vanillylmandelic acid (**VMA**), **metanephrine,** and **normetanephrine** (all breakdown products of the catecholes); urine/serum epi/norepi levels; Hyperglycemia (epi increases glucose, norepi decreases insulin); polycythemia

Tumor localization tests? (5)

CT, MRI, U/S, caval venous sampling for epi/norepi, nuclear scan [^{131}I-MIBG** (metaiodobenzylguanidine) scan]—both sensitive and specific

What is ^{131}I-MIBG?

Metaiodobenzylguanidine

What is the tumor site if epinephrine is elevated?

It must be adrenal or near adrenal (i.e., organs of Zuckerkandl) since nonadrenal tumors lack the capability to methylate norepi to epi

Percentage with malignant tumors?

Adults—10%, children > adults

Preoperative/medical treatment?

Increase intravascular volume with α-blockade (i.e., phenoxybenzamine) and/or α-methyl-1-tyrosine to allow reduction in catecholamine induced vasoconstriction and volume depletion, and β-blocker for reduction of HTN and cardiomegaly; treatment should be started as soon as diagnosis is made

Surgical treatment?

Tumor resection with early ligation of venous drainage (LOWER POSSIBILITY OF CATECHOLAMINE RELEASE→ CRISIS BY TYING OFF DRAINAGE)

Perioperative complications?

- Anesthetic challenge: HTNsive crisis with manipulation (Rx with nitroprusside), hypotension with total removal of the tumor, massive fluid replacement, cardiac arrhythmias (bradycardia, tachycardia)
- Surgical challenge: detecting small extraadrenal tumors/mets.

In the patient with pheo, what must be ruled out?

MEN type II; almost all are BILATERAL

Likely tumor site in the patient with hypertensive crisis with urination?

Bladder pheochromocytoma

Risk of angiography to localize a pheochromocytoma?

May precipitate a hypertensive crisis

What are the organs of Zuckerkandl?

Embryonic chromaffin cells around the abdominal aorta (near the inf. mesenteric art.) that normally atrophy during childhood but are a major site of extraadrenal pheo

CONN'S SYNDROME

What is it?

Hyperaldosteronism; aldosterone is abnormally secreted by an adrenal adenoma/ carcinoma/hyperplasia or by an ovarian tumor

Signs/Sx?	Fatigue, HYPERTENSION, headache, nocturia
What are the two classic clues of Conn's syndrome?	**Hypertension** and **hypokalemia**
Labs?	Increased sodium, decreased potassium (makes sense: aldosterone results in sodium/H_2O retention with loss of K^+), increase in urinary aldosterone, normal or low renin serum levels
Diagnostic tests?	CT, venous sampling for aldosterone, iodocholesterol scanning
What is spironolactone?	Antialdosterone medication
Rx?	Surgical resection

INSULINOMA

What is it?	Insulin-producing tumor arising from Beta cells
Incidence?	#1 islet cell neoplasm; $\frac{1}{2}$ of beta cell tumors of pancreas produce insulin
Risks?	Associated with MEN I syndrome (ppp = pituitary, pancreas, parathyroid tumors)

Signs and symptoms?	Sympathetic discharge
	    Palpitations, diaphoresis, tremulousness,
	        irritability, weakness
	Neuroglycopenic
	    Personality changes, confusion,
	        obtundation, seizures, coma
	Whipple's triad—
	    1. Hypoglycemic symptoms produced by
	        fasting
	    2. Blood Glc <50 mg/dl during
	        symptomatic attack
	    3. Relief of symptoms by administration
	        of glucose

DDx?	Reactive hypoglycemia Functional hypoglycemia with gastrectomy Adrenal insufficiency Hypopituitarism Hepatic insufficiency

Non–islet cell tumor causing hypoglycemia (hemangiopericytoma, fibrosarcoma, leiomyosarcoma, hepatoma, adrenocortical carcinoma)

Surreptitious administration of insulin by self or others (the Sonny Von Bulow case comes to mind!)

Labs?

Glucose and insulin levels during fast; proinsulin levels (if self-injection of insulin is a concern, as insulin injections have no proinsulin)

Diagnostic tests?

1. Fasting hypoglycemia in the presence of inappropriately high levels of insulin
2. 72-hour fast, then check glucose and insulin levels q 6 hr (monitor very closely as patient can have hypoglycemic crisis!)
3. A-gram
4. Percutaneous transhepatic venous catheterization to sample blood along portal and splenic veins to measure insulin and localize tumor
5. Intraoperative ultrasound

Treatment?

Medical—diazoxide to suppress insulin release

Surgical—resection if tumor localized

Prognosis?

≈80% have a benign solitary adenoma that is cured by surgical resection

ZOLLINGER-ELLISON SYNDROME

What is it?

Non–beta islet cell tumor of the pancreas (or other locale) that produces gastrin causing gastric hypersecretion of HCl and GI ulceration; **gastrinoma**

Incidence?

<1% of PUD associated with ZES

Risks?

25% associated with MEN I syndrome

Symptoms?

PUD Sx:
   Burning epigastric pain, relieved by eating or antacids
   Dyspepsia—bloating, nausea, anorexia
Diarrhea (caused by massive acid hypersecretion and destruction of digestive enzymes, NOT intrinsic action of gastrin)

Signs?

Abd tenderness
Guarding/rigidity if perforation

DDx of increased gastrin?	Gastric outlet obstruction Antral G-cell hyperplasia/hyperfunction Postvagotomy Pernicious anemia Atrophic gastritis Short gut syndrome Renal failure
Labs?	Fasting gastrin level Postsecretin challenge gastrin level Calcium (screen for MEN I) Chem 7

Diagnostic tests?	Elevated gastrin
	   NL fasting = 100–200 pg/ml
	   ZES fasting = 200–1000 pg/ml
	Secretin challenge:
	   NL → Decreased gastrin
	   ZES → Increased gastrin
	Basal acid secretion (ZES >15 mEq/hr)
	Hypercalcemia (suspect MEN I)
	UGI
	   Ulcer(s) in usual and **unusual**
	   locations—postduodenal bulb, stomach,
	   jejunum
	   Increased gastric rugal folds
	Selective angio (not always helpful)
	Selective venous sampling

Treatment?	Medical
	   H2 blocker, omeprazole
	Surgical:
	   1. Excision of tumor
	   2. Parietal cell vagotomy
	   3. Total gastrectomy

Prognosis?	Most are malignant, with multicentricity and local spread ≈40% 5-year survival after total gastrectomy
Complications?	Hemorrhage ($\frac{1}{3}$) Perforation Gastric outlet obstruction Intractable pain

THYROID DISEASE

Name three benign lesions of the thyroid	1. Adenomatous goiter 2. Follicular adenoma 3. Hyperfunctioning adenoma

What is Graves' disease? Etiology?

Diffuse goiter with hyperthyroidism, exophthalmos, and pretibial myxedema; it is caused by circulating antibodies that stimulate TSH receptors on follicular cells of the thyroid and cause deregulated production of thyroid hormones

Name 3 treatment modalities for Graves' disease and their relative pro's and con's

1. *Medical Blockade:* iodide, propranolol, propylthiouracil (PTU)
2. *Radioiodide ablation:* Most popular therapy; concern for use during or near pregnancy; many will have secondary hypothyroidism
3. *Surgical resection:* Used if there is also a suspicious nodule, for patients noncompliant with medicines, or patients pregnant or planning pregnancy within a year; complications include hypothyroidism and superior laryngeal/recurrent laryngeal nerve injury

THYROIDITIS

Features of subacute thyroiditis?

Glandular swelling, tender, often follows upper respiratory infection, elevated ESR

Features of Hashimoto's (chronic) thyroiditis?

Firm and rubbery gland, hypothyroid, antibodies elevated

What is the differential diagnosis of a *thyroid nodule?* (7)

1. Adenomatous goiter
2. Adenoma
3. Hyperfunctioning adenoma
4. Cyst
5. Thyroiditis
6. Carcinoma
7. Parathyroid tumor

Name 3 types of nonthyroidal neck masses

1. Inflammatory lesions
2. Congenital lesions; i.e., thyroglossal duct (midline), branchial cleft cyst (lateral)
3. Malignant lesions: lymphoma, metastases

What studies can be used to evaluate a thyroid nodule? (4)

1. Radioiodide or ^{99}Tc scan—hot or cold nodule
2. Ultrasound—solid or cystic
3. Fine needle biopsy—cell pathology
4. Adjunctive blood test
   a. Thyroid panel
   b. Thyroid antibody
   c. TSH

What is meant by a hot versus a cold nodule?

Nodule uptake of IV ^{131}I
HOT: Increased ^{131}I uptake = functioning/
hyperfunctioning
COLD: Decreased ^{131}I uptake =
nonfunctioning nodule

Percentage Malignant _____

Cold thyroid nodule?

10–20% in adults, 50% in children

Sex prevalence?

Males > females

Risk factors?

History of neck irradiation, young > old,
cold nodule, solitary nodule > multiple
nodules

Multinodular mass?

≈1% CA rate

Cystic mass <4 cm diameter?

Almost none; diagnosis by ultrasound or
needle aspiration

What are the pro's and con's of fine needle aspiration?

Safe, cost-effective diagnosis of papillary,
medullary, and anaplastic carcinomas with
less than 5% false negatives; however, **it
cannot accurately distinguish between
benign and malignant follicular tumors**

In evaluating thyroid nodules, what symptoms and signs suggest carcinoma? (7)

1. History of radiation therapy to the neck
2. History of rapid development
3. Vocal cord paralysis
4. Cervical adenopathy
5. Invasion outside thyroid
6. Hard fixed mass in thyroid
7. Elevated serum calcitonin

THYROID CARCINOMA

Name the FOUR main categories of thyroid carcinoma and their relative percentages

1. Papillary carcinoma: 60% (*P*opular =
   *P*apillary)
2. Follicular carcinoma: 20%
3. Medullary carcinoma: 10%
4. Anaplastic/undifferentiated carcinoma:
   10%

Signs and Symptoms?

Mass; most are **euthyroid,** (rarely
hyperfunctioning)

PAPILLARY ADENOCARCINOMA _____

Associated with?

Gardner's syndrome and neck irradiation

Histology?

*P*sammoma bodies (remember, *P* =
*P*sammoma = *P*apillary also, 60% of thyroid
tumors so, *P*apillary = *P*opular)

Route and rate of spread?	Lymphatics (cervical adenopathy); spreads slowly
^{131}I uptake?	Good uptake
10-year survival?	≈80%
Treatment?	Thyroid lobectomy and isthmusectomy, near-total thyroidectomy or total thyroidectomy

FOLLICULAR ADENOCARCINOMA

Nodule consistency?	Rubbery, encapsulated
Route of spread?	Hematogenous, more aggressive than papillary
Male: female ratio?	1:3
^{131}I uptake?	Good uptake
10-year survival?	≈55%
Can diagnosis be made by FNA?	**NO!** Need tissue structure for diagnosis
Treatment?	Near total thyroidectomy

MEDULLARY CARCINOMA

Associated with?	Multiple endocrine neoplasia type II; autosomal dominant genetic transmission
Histology?	A*m*yloid. (A**M**yloid = **M**edullary)
Secretes what?	Calcitonin
Route and rate of spread?	Lymphatic; relatively rapid spread
^{131}I uptake?	Poor uptake
Prognosis?	10-year survival is 50%; however, the cure rate is 95% when occult tumors are found in MEN family members being screened for elevated calcitonin; if detected when clinically palpable, the cure rate is <20%
Treatment?	Total thyroidectomy and median lymph node dissection

ANAPLASTIC CARCINOMA

Gender preference?	Female > male
Histology?	Giant, spindle, small, or squamous cells
^{131}I uptake?	Very poor uptake

Prognosis?	Dismal, as most patients are at stage IV at presentation; survival past 2 years is rare
Describe the blood supply to the thyroid	1. Paired superior thyroid arteries from the external carotids 2. Paired inferior thyroid arteries from the thyrocervical trunks 3. Paired superior, middle, and inferior thyroid veins
What paired arteries supply all four parathyroids?	The inferior thyroid arteries (not 100%!)
What paired nerves must be carefully identified and how?	The **recurrent laryngeal nerves** are found in the tracheoesophageal grooves and dive into the cricothyroid groove; damage to these nerves paralyzes laryngeal abductors and causes hoarseness
What other nerve is at risk and what are the symptoms?	**Superior laryngeal nerve**—opera singers are unable to hit the high pitches—thus the patient will have a deeper and quieter voice
What laboratory value must be followed postoperatively?	Decreased **calcium** (and increased phosphorus levels) secondary to parathyroid damage; during lobectomy, the parathyroids must be spared and their blood supply protected; if blood supply is compromised intraoperatively, they can be autografted into the sternocleomastoid muscle or forearm
DDx of postoperative dyspnea?	1. Neck hematoma→remove sutures and clot at *bedside* 2. *Bilateral* recurrent laryngeal nerve damage
What is a "lateral aberrant rest" of the thyroid?	A misnomer! It is *papillary* CA of a lymph node from a metastasis!

HYPERPARATHYROIDISM (↑PTH)

Define 1° ↑PTH	Increased secretion of PTH by parathyroid gland(s) (see etiologies below)
Define 2° ↑PTH	Increase in serum PTH due to **renal failure** and constant Ca^{2+} wasting
Define 3° ↑PTH	Persistent ↑PTH due to **refractory hyperplasia** caused by 2° ↑PTH (after serum Ca^{2+} is corrected, Ca^{2+} fails to regulate PTH secretion)

Etiologies of 1° ↑PTH and percentages? (3)

Adenoma (≈85%)
Hyperplasia (≈15%)
Carcinoma (≈1%)

What is the incidence of 1° ↑PTH in the U.S.?

≈1/1000

Risk factors for 1° ↑PTH (2)

Family Hx; irradiation

Signs/Sx of 1° ↑PTH? (14)

"Bones, groans, and psychiatric overtones"; due to hypercalcemia
BONES: Bone pain (actually rare)
GROANS: Muscle pain and weakness, pancreatitis, nephrolithiasis, gout.
Ψ OVERTONES: Depression, anorexia, lethargy, anxiety
OTHERS: Polydipsia, wgt loss, **constipation,** HTN (10%), polyuria.

Diagnosis of 1° ↑PTH? (4)

LABS—Hypercalcemia, ↑PTH levels, ↓phosphorus, ↑*chloride*

How many of the glands are affected by
    Hyperplasia?
    Adenoma?
    Carcinoma?

4
1
1

Differential Dx? (15)

Causes (DDx) of hypercalcemia:
"C.H.I.M.P.A.N.Z.E.E.S."
Calcium↑:
Hyperparathyroidism (1°/2°/3°)
Hyperthyroidism
Immobility/**I**atrogenic (thiazide diuretics)
Mets/**M**ilk alkali syndrome (rare)
Paget's disease (bone)
Addison's disease/**A**cromegaly
Neoplasm (colon, lung, breast, prostate, multiple myeloma)
Zollinger-Ellison syndrome
Excessive vitamin D
Excessive vitamin A
Sarcoid

Primary treatment (1° ↑PTH)?

MEDICAL—IV fluids, furosemide *NOT* thiazide diuretics

Definitive treatment (1° ↑PTH)?

Neck exploration removing abnormal parathyroid glands and leaving at least 50 mg of normal parathyroid tissue (often placed in the forearm)

What must be ruled out in the patient with 1° ↑PTH?	MEN type I and MEN type IIa
Usual # of parathyroid glands?	Four
Percentage with a parathyroid gland in the mediastinum?	≈1%
Blood supply to parathyroid glands?	Inferior thyroid vessels
Cell type that produces PTH?	Chief cells
What is the 33 to 1 rule?	Patients with 1° HPTH have a ratio of serum $[Cl^-]$ to [phosphate] ≥33
If at operation you find only 3 parathyroid glands, where can the 4th one be hiding?	Thyroid gland Thymus/mediastinum Carotid sheath Tracheoesophageal groove
What carcinoma is commonly associated with hypercalcemia?	*Breast CA* mets

MULTIPLE ENDOCRINE NEOPLASIA (MEN)

Inheritance?	Autosomal dominant (but with a significant degree of variation in penetrance)

MEN TYPE I _____

Common eponym?	Wermer's syndrome (Think, **W**ermer = **W**inner = type **1**)
Most common abnormalities, their incidences and symptoms? (3)	**PPP:** **P**arathyroid hyperplasia (≈90%**) • Hypercalcemia **P**ancreatic islet cell tumors (≈⅔) • Gastrinoma: Zollinger-Ellison syndrome (½) • Insulinoma (20%) **P**ituitary tumors (≈⅔) —optic defects Think: type 1 = **p**rimary, **p**rimary, **p**rimary = **PPP** = **p**arathyroid, **p**ancreas, **p**ituitary

MEN TYPE IIA _____

Common eponym?	Sipple's syndrome (Think, **S**ipple's = **S**econd = type **2**)

Most common abnormalities, their incidences and symptoms? (3)

MPH:
*M*edullary thyroid carcinoma (**100%)
• Calcitonin secreted
• Dx with Pentagastrin stimulation test
*P*heochromocytoma (>⅓)
• Catecholamine excess
Parathyroid hyperplasia (≈¼)
*H*yperparathyroidism (about ½)
• Hypercalcemia
Think: type 2 = 2 MPH or 2 miles per hour = **MPH** = **m**edullary, **p**heochromocytoma, **h**yperparathyroid

MEN TYPE IIB

Most common abnormalities, their incidences and symptoms? (4)

MMMP
Mucosal neuromas (100%)
In the nasopharynx, oropharynx, larynx, and conjunctiva
Medullary thyroid carcinoma (≈85%)—more aggressive than in MEN IIa
Marfanoid body habitus (long/lanky)
Pheochromocytoma (≈50%) and found bilaterally**

32
Spleen and Splenectomy

Arterial supply to spleen?
Arterial supply is from the splenic artery, a branch of the celiac trunk, and the short gastric arteries that arise from the gastroepiploic arteries and splenic artery

What percentage of people have accessory spleens?
About 1 in 5

What is the spleen's claim to infamy?
The **spleen** is the **most common** intraabdominal organ injured in **blunt trauma**

What is "delayed splenic rupture"?
Subcapsular hematomas may rupture at a later time after blunt trauma causing "delayed splenic rupture"; most commonly rupture about 2 weeks after the injury and present with shock/abdominal pain

Signs/Sx of rupture?
Hemoperitoneum + Kehr's sign (referred pain to the tip of the left shoulder) and LUQ pain/abdominal pain (**blood can be a peritoneal irritant after several hours**)

Dx?
CT**, ultrasound, exploratory laparotomy

Rx?
Nonoperative in a stable patient with an **isolated** splenic injury without hilar involvement or complete rupture; otherwise laparotomy and if possible a splenic salvage operation (with wrapping/aid of topical hemostatic agents), otherwise splenectomy; VAST majority of pediatric patients undergo nonoperative Rx for blunt spleen injury! (Expeditious splenectomy in multiply injured adult trauma patient)

Other indications for splenectomy?
For control/staging of disease/ hypersplenism
    Gaucher's disease
    Splenic vein thrombosis
    Sickle cell disease

Thrombocytopenia associated with drug
 abuse
Spherocytosis
Lymphomas (esp. Hodgkin's disease)
ITP
TTP
Splenic tumors
Splenic trauma
Felty's syndrome
Lymphoproliferative disorders (i.e., NHL,
 CLL)
Hairy cell leukemia
Thalassemia major

Is G6PD deficiency an indication for splenectomy?

NO (typical board question)

Postsplenectomy complications?

Thrombocytosis (Rx with **ASA** if platelet count is ≥1 million), subphrenic abscess, gastric dilation, and *overwhelming postsplenectomy sepsis* (**OPSS**)

What is OPSS?

Increased susceptibility to fulminant bacteremia, meningitis, or pneumonia due to loss of splenic function

What is the typical presentation of OPSS?

Nausea, vomiting, and headache, in an individual with a febrile upper respiratory illness, followed by confusion, shock, and coma with death ensuing within 24 hr in over half

Common organisms in OPSS?

**Encapsulated: #1 *Streptococcus pneumoniae* accounts >50% of cases; also meningococcus, *H. influenzae,* and *E. coli* (*Note:* these organisms are normally removed by a functioning splenic reticular

Prevention of OPSS?

Prophylactic penicillin in the immunosuppressed and the need for immediate medical care should a febrile illness develop; also vaccinations for **pneumococcus,** HIB, and polyvalent meningococcal vaccines

Why is an NG tube necessary after splenectomy?

To prevent gastric distention which can blow out suture ties used to control the short gastric vessels

What lab tests are abnormal after splenectomy?

WBC count increases by 50% over baseline for about a week postop; Marked **thrombocytosis** occurs; Peripheral smear will show Pappenheimer/Howell-Jolly bodies; low levels of opsonins produced in the spleen

When to Rx thrombocytopenia?

When > million platelets—Rx with aspirin

Common cause of splenic vein thrombosis?

Pancreatitis

What opsonins are produced by the spleen?

Tuftsin, properdin

Common cause of ISOLATED gastric varices?

Splenic vein thrombosis

Who gets hyposplenism?

Patients with ulcerative colitis

What vaccinations should every patient with a splenectomy get?

Vaccinations against

1. Pneumococcus
2. Meningococcus
3. *Haemophilus influenzae* type b

Define hypersplenism

1. Hyperfunctioning spleen
2. Documented loss of blood elements (WBC, hct, platelets)
3. Large spleen (splenomegaly)
4. Hyperactive bone marrow (trying to keep up with the loss of blood elements!)

33
Surgically Correctable HTN

What is it?   Hypertension caused by conditions that are amendable to surgical correction

What percentage of patients with hypertension have a surgically correctable cause?   About 7%

What are the diseases that cause HTN and are surgically correctable?

Renal artery stenosis
Pheochromocytoma
Unilateral renal parenchymal disease
Cushing's syndrome
Conn's syndrome (primary hyperaldosteronism)
Hyperparathyroidism/Hyperthyroidism
Coarctation of the aorta
Cancer
Neuroblastoma
Increased intracranial pressure

What is the formula for pressure?   Pressure = flow × resistance or $P = F \times R$ (Think, **P**ower **F**o**R**ward); thus, an increase in flow and/or resistance results in an increase in pressure

NEUROBLASTOMA

What is it?   Embryonal tumor of neural crest origin; seen in children

Average age at Dx?   **50% by 2 yr**
90% by 8 yr

Sx?   **Vary by tumor location—anemia, failure to thrive, wgt loss and poor nutritional status with advanced disease**

Signs?   **Asymptomatic abdominal mass (palpable in 50%), respiratory distress (mediastinal tumors), Horner's syndrome (upper chest or neck tumors), proptosis (with orbital metastases), subcutaneous tumor nodules, HTN (20–35%)**

| What causes HTN in neuroblastoma? | Increased catecholamines |

PHEOCHROMOCYTOMA

| What is it? | Tumor of the adrenal medulla and other similar tissues (e.g., sympathetic ganglion) that produces catecholamines (epi, norepi, dopamine) |
| What causes the HTN in pheochromocytoma? | Increased catecholamines |

RENAL ARTERY STENOSIS

What is it?	Stenosis of the renal artery resulting in decreased perfusion of the juxtaglomerular apparatus and subsequent activation of the aldosterone-renin-angiotensin system
Sx/signs?	Most are asymptomatic, but may have headache, *diastolic* **HTN,** flank bruits (present in 50%), and decreased renal function; *Note:* ≈7% of essential hypertensives also have flank bruits
What causes of HTN in renal artery stenosis?	Increased renin→angiotensin/aldosterone

COARCTATION OF THE AORTA

| What is it? | Narrowing of thoracic aorta ± intraluminal "shelf" (infolding of the media), usually found near ductus/ligamentum arteriosum |
| What causes the HTN in coarctation? | Increase in resistance to flow to distal body and thus increased flow to upper body |

HYPERPARATHYROIDISM (↑PTH)

Define ↑PTH.	Increased secretion of PTH
What percentage of patients with hyperparathyroidism have hypertension?	About 10%
What causes the hypertension in hyperparathyroidism?	Hypercalcemia

CONN'S SYNDROME

What is it?

Hyperaldosteronism. Aldosterone is abnormally secreted by an adrenal adenoma/carcinoma/hyperplasia or by an ovarian tumor

What are the two classic clues of Conn's syndrome?

Hypertension and **hypokalemia**

What causes the hypertension in Conn's syndrome?

Hypervolemia

CUSHING'S SYNDROME

What is it?

Excessive cortisol production.

What percentage have hypertension?

>75%!

What causes the hypertension in Cushing's syndrome?

Hypervolemia

INCREASED INTRACRANIAL PRESSURE

What causes the hypertension in increased ICP?

The Cushing's response (reflex)—**hypertension** and **bradycardia**

CANCER

What causes the hypertension in cancer?

Paraneoplastic syndromes

34
Sarcomas and Lymphomas

SARCOMA

What is it?	Soft tissue tumors; derived from mesoderm
How common?	1% of malignant tumors; incidence peaks under age 15

Name the sarcoma of

Fat	Liposarcoma
Smooth muscle	Leiomyosarcoma
Histiocyte	Malignant fibrous histiocytoma
Striated muscle	Rhabdomyosarcoma
Vascular endothelium	Angiosarcoma
Fibroblast	Fibrosarcoma
Lymph vessel	Lymphangiosarcoma
Peripheral nerve	Malignant neurilemmoma or schwannoma
AIDS	Kaposi's sarcoma

Signs/Sx?	Soft tissue mass, pain from compression of adjacent structures
How do most sarcomas metastasize?	Via blood (hematogenously)
Most common two in adults?	Liposarcoma (20%) Fibrous histiocytoma
Most common two in children?	Rhabdomyosarcoma (about ½) Fibrosarcoma (20%)
Most common metastasis to where? How?	**Lungs** via hematogenous route
Most common type to metastasize to lymph node?	Malignant fibrous histiocytoma
Most frequent type formed in retroperitoneum?	Liposarcoma
How do sarcomas locally invade?	Usually along anatomic planes such as fascia, vessels, etc.

Diagnosis?

Extensive imaging workup—MRI is superior to CT at distinguishing the tumor from adjacent structures;

<3 cm mass: excisional biopsy

>3 cm incisional biopsy, cxr, chest CT

What is a *pseudocapsule* and what is its importance?

It is the outer layer of a sarcoma that represents compressed malignant cells. Microscopic extensions of tumor cells invade through the pseudocapsule into adjacent structures. Thus, definitive therapy must include a wide margin of resection to account for this phenomenon and not just be "shelled-out" like a benign growth.

Prognosis?

Histologic grade of the primary lesion is the most important factor!

Treatment?

Radical surgery (i.e., amputation) produces fewer local recurrences than local resection; however, conservative surgery with radiation therapy produces equal results to those of radical surgery; combined therapy local recurrence rate: about $\frac{1}{4}$

Rx pulmonary metastasis?

Surgical resection for isolated lesions

LYMPHOMA

What treatments are used for low vs. advanced stage Hodgkin's lymphoma?

Low stage: radiotherapy

Advanced stage: chemotherapy

Diagnosis?

Cervical or axillary node excisional biopsy

What is a staging laparotomy for Hodgkin's lymphoma?

It is a laparotomy to distinguish between advanced and low-stage disease to design proper therapy as above. It includes splenectomy and extensive biopsies of splenic hilar, celiac, mesenteric, porta hepatis, paraaortic, and iliac lymph nodes. The liver is biopsied, and if the patient is of childbearing years the ovaries are marked with metallic clips and then tacked behind the uterus (oophoropexy) for protection from radiation fields.

Is staging laparotomy indicated for non-Hodgkin's lymphoma?

Rarely, as most patients present with systemic disease and will need combination radiation and chemotherapy

Rx for gastric lymphoma?

Gastric lymphoma requires resection and staging biopsies

Rx for intestinal lymphoma?

Resect with removal of draining lymph nodes

What is stage A Hodgkin's?

Asymptomatic = stage A

What is stage B Hodgkin's?

Symptomatic; wgt loss, fever, night sweats, etc.
Think, stage $B = B$ad

Define for Hodgkin's:
  Stage I

Single lymph node region

  Stage II

Two or more lymph node regions on **same side of diaphragm**

  Stage III

Involvement on **both** sides of the diaphragm

  Stage IV

Diffuse and/or disseminated involvement

Percentage with Hodgkin's cured?

Approximately 80%

4 histopathologic types of Hodgkin's?

1. Nodular sclerosing (most common)
2. Mixed cellularity
3. Lymphocyte predominant
4. Lymphocyte depleted

35
Melanoma

What is it?

Neoplastic disorder produced by malignant transformation of the melanocyte; melanocytes are derived from neural crest cells and can be found anywhere on the body

Incidence?

almost all are white

Characteristics suggestive of melanoma?

Darkening of a pigmented lesion, development of pigmented satellite lesions, irregular margins or surface elevations, notching, recent or rapid enlargement, erosion or ulceration of surface, pruritus

Risk factors?

Giant congenital nevi, family history, white, ultraviolet radiation (sun), multiple dysplastic nevi.

Regional factors?

Men get more lesions on the trunk; women get them on the extremities

Unusual locations include noncutaneous regions such as mucous membranes of the vulva/vagina, anorectum, esophagus, and choroidal layer of the eye

Histological types?

1. *Superficial spreading melanoma*—occurs in both sun-exposed and nonexposed areas; $\frac{2}{3}$ overall
2. *Lentigo maligna melanoma*—spindle-shaped malignant cells that are junctional in location; 10%; found usually in elderly on the head or neck
3. *Acral lentiginous melanoma*—palms, soles, subungual areas, and mucous membranes; 10%
4. *Nodular melanoma*—vertical growth predominates; 15%

What is lentigo?

A brown reddish flat spot on the skin caused by excess melanin, which can degenerate into a cancer

What type of melanoma arises in a Hutchinson's freckle?

Lentigo maligna melanoma

Prognosis?

Depth of invasion is the most important factor; other factors include pathologic stage, ulceration, surgical treatment, and primary site location.

Superficial spreading and lentigo maligna have a better prognosis because they have a longer horizontal phase of growth and are thus diagnosed at an earlier stage.

Nodular has the worst prognosis because it grows predominantly vertically and metastasizes earlier.

Clark's classification (microstaging of tumor)
  I?

I. Tumor confined to epidermis—basically 0% 5-year recurrence rate

  II?

II. Tumor invades papillary dermis—<5% 5-year recurrence rate

  III?

III. Tumor cells up to the junction of papillary and reticular dermis—$\frac{1}{3}$ 5-year recurrence rate

  IV?

IV. Invasion into reticular dermis—about $\frac{2}{3}$ 5-year recurrence rate

  V?

V. Invasion into subcutaneous fat—$\frac{3}{4}$ 5-year recurrence rate

Breslow classification (microstaging of tumor)?

Staging by actually measuring the depth of the lesion:

<0.76 mm thickness has >90% cure with simple excision
>4.0 mm has at least an 80% risk of local recurrence or metastasis in 5 years

How does one remember Breslow versus Clarke's classifications?

Simply think, Bres**low** = low = depth by measurement

Which tumor staging is more accurate in predicting survival?

The Breslow classification—a more consistent measure of tumor thickness

TNM (Tumor-nodes-metastasis) staging
  I?
  II?

Stages I–IV
(abbreviated/simplified)
I: Local disease, tumor < 1.5 mm
II: Local disease, tumor > 1.5 mm, or any size tumor with satellite lesions within 2 cm of primary; no nodes, no mets

III?	III:
	a. Any tumor size
	b. + nodes of 1 regional node station
	c. No mets
IV?	IV: a. Any tumor, any nodes, plus mets
	b. Any tumor, no mets, nodes from more than 1 station or large/fixed nodes

Common sites of metastasis?

#1 Nodes local and distant skin recurrence, lung, liver, bone, heart and brain; melanoma has a specific attraction for small bowel mucosa and distant cutaneous sites, brain mets common cause of death

Metastatic routes?

Both lymphatic and hematogenous

Dx/Rx?

Early diagnosis and treatment is crucial Excisional biopsy (complete removal leaving only normal tissue) or incisioned biopsy for very large lesions.

Nodes?

Although further study is needed and underway, there is general agreement that tumors <0.76 mm thick have a low incidence of involved nodes and appear not to benefit from nodal dissection, and tumors >4.0 mm thick have little to gain from node dissection as most already have systemic disease. Remember, lymph node dissection is fraught with morbidity—lymphedema etc! Node dissection for intermediate-thickness melanoma under debate

Mets?

In some cases, surgical resection of solitary metastatic lesions may relieve symptoms (i.e., intestinal met) and may prolong disease-free survival

Rx intestinal mets?

Surgical resection to prevent bleeding/obstruction

Need how much of a surgical margin?

By depth of invasion:
0.5 cm margin if melanoma in situ
1 cm margin if 1 mm thick
2 cm margin if 2 mm thick
2–3 cm margin if >2 mm thick
(or in other words: add 1 cm margin for every mm of depth)

Can melanoma cross the placenta?

Yes

36
Surgical Intensive Care

INTENSIVE CARE UNIT FORMULAE/TERMS YOU SHOULD KNOW

C.O.?

Cardiac **O**utput = HR (heart rate) × SV (stroke volume)

PCWP?

"Wedge pressure"; **p**ost **c**apillary **w**edge **p**ressure

C.I.?

Cardiac **i**ndex = C.O./BSA (body surface area)

S.V.?

Stroke **V**olume = the amount of blood pumped out of the ventricle each beat; simply, end diastolic volume minus the end systolic volume or

$$CO/HR$$

Anion gap?

$Na^+ - (Cl^- + HCO_3^-)$

SVR?

Systemic vascular resistance =

$$\frac{BP - CVP}{CO} \times 80$$

(remember, P = FXR, **P**ower **Fo**R**ward; and calculating resistance: R = P/F and thus the above)

PVR?

Pulmonary vascular resistance =

$$\frac{PA - LA}{CO} \times 80$$

(PA is pulmonary artery pressure and LA is left atrial or PCWP pressure, again remember **P**ower **Fo**R**ward, **R = P/F**)

Arterial oxygen content?

Hemaglobin × O_2 saturation (SaO_2)

Do$_2$?

Oxygen delivery =
C.O. × (hemaglobin × Sao_2)

180

What factors can increase oxygen delivery?

Increase C.O. by increasing S.V. and/or HR, increase oxygen content by either increasing the hemaglobin and/or increase Sao_2

What is mixed venous oxygen saturation?

Svo_2; simply, the O_2 saturation of the blood in the right ventricle; an indirect measure of peripheral oxygen supply and demand

FENa?

Fractional excretion of sodium

$$\frac{U_{Na^+} \times S_{cr}}{S_{Na^+} \times U_{cr}} \times 100$$

To remember, think of the U.S. as #1 or on top, thus, $U \times S$ is in the numerator. Then to define the subscripts remember U.S. again or **U** **S**odium and therefore, $U_{Na^+} \times S_{CR}$; for the denominator switch everything, or $S_{Na^+} \times U_{CR}$

Prerenal FENa value?

<1.0; renal failure due to decreased renal blood flow (cardiogenic, hypovolemia, arterial obstruction etc)

What is the formula for flow/ pressure/resistance?

Remember **P**ower **F**o**R**ward:
Pressure = **F**low × **R**esistance

What is the 10 for 0.08 rule of acid-base?

For every increase of $PaCO_2$ by 10 mm Hg, the pH falls by 0.08.

What is the 40, 50, 60 for 70, 80, 90 rule for O_2 sats?

A PaO_2 of **40, 50, 60** corresponds roughly to an O_2 sat of **70, 80, 90,** respectively

One liter of O_2 via nasal cannula raises FiO_2 by how much?

About 3–4%

Pure respiratory acidosis?

Low pH (acidosis), nl (or high with compensation) bicarb, and **increased $PaCO_2$**

Pure respiratory alkalosis?

High pH (alkalosis), nl (or low with compensation) bicarb, **and decreased $PaCO_2$**

Pure metabolic acidosis?

Low pH, nl (or low with compensation) $PaCO_2$, and **low bicarb**

Pure metabolic alkalosis?

High pH, nl (or high with compensation) $PaCO_2$, and **high bicarb**

MOF?

Multiple organ failure

SICU DRUGS

DOPAMINE

Site of Action and Effect

Low dose (1–3 μg/kg/min)?	++ Dopa agonist; **renal vasodilation** (A.K.A. "renal dose dopamine")
Intermediate dose (2–5 μg/kg/ min)?	+ Alpha, ++ beta; positive inotropy and some vasoconstriction
High dose (>5 μg/kg/min)?	+++ Alpha agonist; marked afterload increase due to arteriolar vasoconstriction

DOBUTAMINE

Site of action?	+++ $Beta_1$ agonist, ++ $beta_2$
Effect?	↑ Inotropy; ↑ chronotropy

ISOPROTERENOL

Site of action?	+++ $Beta_1$ and $beta_2$ agonist
Effect?	↑ Inotropy; ↑ chronotropy; (+ vasodilation of skeletal and mesenteric vascular beds)

EPINEPHRINE

Site of action?	$Alpha_1$, $alpha_2$, $beta_1$, and $beta_2$ agonist
Effect?	↑ Inotropy; ↑ chronotropy; not much change in blood pressure due to peripheral vasodilation

NOREPINEPHRINE

Site of action?	$Alpha_1$, $alpha_2$, and $beta_1$ agonist
Effect?	↑ Inotropy; ↑ chronotropy; ++ increase in blood pressure

NITROGLYCERINE (NTG)

Site of action?	+++ Venodilation; + arteriolar dilation
Effect?	Increased venous capacitance & decreased preload

SODIUM NITROPRUSSIDE (SNP)

Site of action?	+++ Venodilation; +++ arteriolar dilation
Effect?	Deceased preload; decreased afterload (allowing blood pressure titration)

INTENSIVE CARE PHYSIOLOGY

Define _____

Preload?	Preload: the load on the heart muscle that stretches it to end-diastolic volume (end-diastolic pressure)
Afterload?	Afterload: the load on the heart muscle at the beginning of systole (end-diastolic pressure plus aortic diastolic pressure)
Contractility?	Contractility: the force of heart muscle contraction at a certain preload and afterload
Compliance?	Compliance: the distensibility of the heart by the preload

What is the clinical significance of the steep slope of the Starling curve relating end-diastolic volume to systolic pressure?	It demonstrates the importance of preload in determining cardiac output.
What factors can affect cardiac compliance?	The most common factors thought to lower compliance: positive-pressure ventilation, myocardial ischemia, myocardial edema, ventricular hypertrophy, and pericardial tamponade
What factors influence the oxygen content of whole blood?	Oxygen content is composed **largely** of that oxygen bound to hemoglobin, and is thus determined by the hemoglobin concentration and the arterial oxygen saturation; the partial pressure of oxygen dissolved in plasma plays a minor role.
What determines the oxygen delivery to the tissues?	The oxygen content of whole blood and the cardiac output
What factors influence mixed venous oxygen saturation?	Oxygen delivery (hemoglobin concentration, arterial oxygen saturation, cardiac output) and oxygen extraction
What lab for tissue ischemia is based on the shift from aerobic to anaerobic metabolism?	Serum lactate levels

Define _____

Dead space?	Dead space: that part of the inspired air that will not participate in gas exchange; it includes the anatomic dead space (the gas in

the large airways/ET tube not in contact with capillaries) and the physiologic dead space (the alveolar gas that does not equilibrate with capillary blood). Think: space = air

Shunt fraction?

Shunt fraction: that fraction of pulmonary venous blood that did not participate in gas exchange. Think: shunt = blood

What causes increased dead space?

Overventilation (emphysema, excessive PEEP) or underperfusion (pulmonary embolus, low cardiac output)

What is the physiologic effect of increasing dead space ventilation?

Progressive hypoxemia and hypercapnia

What causes increased shunt fraction?

Underventilation (pneumonia, pulmonary edema, respiratory distress syndrome, mucous plugging) or overperfusion (loss of pulmonary vascular autoregulation as in massive pulmonary embolus)

What is the physiologic effect of increasing shunt fraction?

Initially progressive hypoxemia, then late hypercapnia

At high shunt fractions what is the effect of increasing FiO_2 on arterial PO_2?

At high shunt fractions (>50%) changes in FiO_2 have almost **no effect** on arterial PO_2, as the blood that does "see" the O_2 is already at MAXIMAL O_2 absorption and thus, increasing the FiO_2 has no effect; (FiO_2 can be minimized to prevent oxygen toxicity)

At what concentration does O_2 toxicity occur?

>FiO_2 of 60% × 48 hours, thus try to keep FiO_2 below 50% at all times

What are the main causes of carbon dioxide retention?

Hypoventilation, increased dead space ventilation, and increased carbon dioxide production as in hypermetabolic states

Why are carbohydrates minimized in the diet/TPN of patients having difficulty with hypercapnia?

The respiratory quotient (RQ) is the ratio of carbon dioxide production to oxygen consumption, and is highest for carbohydrates (1.0) and lowest for fats (0.7); by minimizing carbohydrate consumption the carbon dioxide production at any metabolic rate is minimized

HEMODYNAMIC MONITORING

Why are indwelling arterial lines used for blood pressure monitoring in critically ill patients?

Because of the need for frequent measurements, the inaccuracy of frequently repeated cuff measurements, the inaccuracy of cuff measurements in hypotension, and the need for frequent blood sampling

Pressures obtained from a Swan-Ganz catheter?

CVP/RAP, PA pressures, PCWP, CO, PVR

What is PCWP?

Pulmonary capillary wedge pressure: Essentially equivalent to left ventricular end diastolic pressure (LVEDP) = left atrial pressure (LAP), i.e., left heart preload

What is the primary use of the pulmonary capillary wedge pressure?

As a measure of left atrial pressure; only when ventricular compliance is normal and unchanging is the wedge pressure an accurate estimate of left ventricular end diastolic pressure, and thus preload

At what point in the respiratory cycle are pulmonary artery pressure readings most useful?

At end expiration, when intrathoracic pressure equals atmospheric pressure, the pulmonary artery pressure reflects the transmural pressure

In which clinical situations is pulmonary capillary wedge pressure not an accurate estimate of preload?

Pulmonary disease such as adult respiratory distress syndrome or pulmonary hypertension, valvular heart disease, ischemic heart disease with a noncompliant ventricle

What are possible sources of error in the thermodilution measurement of CO?

Tricuspid insufficiency, intracardiac shunts, prolonged injection times, catheter occlusion

MECHANICAL VENTILATION

Define

IMV?

Intermittent mandatory ventilation; mode with intermittent ventilations at a predetermined rate and patients can also breathe on their own above the mandatory rate **without** help from the ventilator

A-C?

Assist/control ventilation; mode in which the ventilator delivers a breath when the patient initiates a breath, or the ventilator "assists" the patient to breathe; if the patient does not initiate a breath, the ventilator takes "control" and delivers a breath at a predetermined rate

What are the effects of positive pressure ventilation in a patient with hypovolemia or low lung compliance?

If the patient is hypovolemic then venous return is decreased and cardiac output is decreased. If the patient has stiff lungs requiring high intrathoracic pressures then venous return is decreased, pulmonary artery pressure is increased, left ventricular filling is decreased, cardiac output falls, and the risk of right heart failure increases.

Side effects of increasing levels of PEEP?

Barotrauma (injury to airway = pneumothorax), decreased CO due to decreased preload

What are typical initial ventilator settings?

Mode: intermittent mandatory ventilation or assist control
Tidal volume: 12 ml/kg
Ventilator rate: 12 breaths/min
FiO2: 100% and wean down
   PEEP: most use 5 cm H_2O as a "physiologic" PEEP
   **From these parameters change according to blood gas analysis

What clinical situations cause an increase in airway resistance?

Airway or endotracheal tube obstruction, bronchospasm, A.R.D.S.

What clinical situations cause a decrease in respiratory compliance?

Pneumothorax, atelectasis, pneumonia, pulmonary edema, alveolar air trapping

What are the presumed advantages of positive end expiratory pressure (PEEP)?

Prevention of alveolar collapse and atelectasis, improved gas exchange, increased pulmonary compliance, decreased shunt fraction

What are the possible disadvantages of PEEP?

Decreased cardiac output especially in the setting of hypovolemia, decreased gas exchange, and compliance with high levels of PEEP, fluid retention, increased intracranial pressure, barotrauma

What parameters must be evaluated in deciding if a patient is ready to be extubated?

Gas exchange ($PaO_2/PaCO_2$ on blood gas), tidal volume, minute ventilation, negative inspiratory pressure

Possible source of fever in a patient with a NG tube or nasal endotracheal tube?

SINUSITIS, Dx by sinus films

37
Vascular Surgery

GENERAL

Atherosclerosis: what is it?

A diffuse disease process in arteries; atheromas containing cholesterol and lipid form within the intima and inner media, often accompanied by ulcerations and smooth muscle hyperplasia

Risk factors for atherosclerosis?

Hypertension, smoking, diabetes mellitus, family hx, hypercholesterolemia, obesity, and sedentary lifestyle

Common site of plaque formation in arteries?

Branch points

PERIPHERAL VASCULAR DISEASE

What is it?

Occlusive atherosclerotic disease in lower extremities

Symptoms?

Intermittent claudication, rest pain, impotence, sensorimotor impairment, tissue loss

What is intermittent claudication?

Pain and/or cramping of the lower extremity, usually the calf muscle, after walking a specific distance; then the pain/cramping resolves after stopping a specific amount of time while standing; this is all reproducible

What is rest pain?

Pain in the foot, usually over the distal metatarsels; this pain arises at rest! classically at night, awaking the patient

What classically resolves the rest pain?

Hanging the foot over the side of the bed or standing—gravity affords some extra flow to the ischemic areas

How does one differentiate vascular causes of claudication from nonvascular causes such as neurogenic claudication or arthritis?

HISTORY, in the vast majority of patients, and noninvasive tests; remember, vascular claudication appears after a specific distance and resolves after a specific time of rest while standing—this is not so with most other forms of claudication

DDx of lower extremity claudication?

Neurogenic (nerve entrapment/discs, etc.), arthritis, coarctation of the aorta, popliteal artery syndrome, chronic compartment syndromes, neuromas, anemia

Signs of PVD?

Decreased or absent pulses, bruits, muscular atrophy, decreased hair growth, thick toenails, tissue necrosis/ulcers/infection

What is ABI?

The ankle to brachial index (ABI); simply, the ratio of the systolic blood pressure at the ankle to the systolic blood pressure at the arm (brachial artery) A:B; ankle pressure taken with Doppler; the ABI is noninvasive

What ABIs are associated with normals, claudicators, and rest pain?

Normal ABI ≥ 1.0
Claudicator ABI = <0.7
Rest pain ABI <0.4

Who gets false ABI readings?

Those with calcified arteries, especially diabetics

Prior to surgery for chronic PVD what diagnostic test will every patient get?

A-gram maps disease and allows for best treatment option (i.e., angioplasty vs. surgical bypass vs. endarterectomy)

Indications for surgical Rx in PVD?

1. Rest pain
2. Tissue necrosis or threatened limb
3. Severe claudication refractory to conservative Rx and that affects quality of life/livelihood

Treatment for claudication?

Vast, vast majority—conservative Rx; this includes *exercise*, stop smoking*, Rx HTN, diet

Risk of limb loss with claudication?

5% limb loss at 5 years (think: 5 in 5)

Risk of limb loss with rest pain?

>50% will have amputation of the limb at some point

In the patient with PVD one must worry about what preoperatively?

Cardiac status, as most patients with PVD have coronary artery disease and about 20% have an AAA; MI most common cause of postoperative death after PVD Rx

What is LeRiche syndrome?

Impotence, buttock claudication, gluteus muscle atrophy due to occlusive disease of the iliacs/distal Ao

What are the Rx options for severe PVD?

1. Surgical graft bypass
2. Angioplasty—balloon dilation
3. Endarterectomy—remove diseased intima and media

Autologous versus prosthetic grafts?

Autologous (usually saphenous vein graft) have better long-term patency rates than prosthetic material, but removing the saphenous vein does not allow future saphenous vein coronary artery bypass

ACUTE ARTERIAL OCCLUSION

What is it?

Acute occlusion of an artery, usually by embolization; other causes include acute thrombosis of atheromatous lesion, vascular trauma

Classic signs/Sx of acute arterial occlusion?

6 P's: pain, paralysis, pallor, paresthesia, polar (some say poikilothermia—you pick), pulselessness (*you *must* know these!)

Immediate preoperative management?

1. Anticoagulate with heparin IV (bolus followed by constant infusion)
2. A-gram

Rx options?

1. Surgical embolectomy via cutdown and Fogarty balloon
2. Thrombectomy
3. Surgical bypass

What is a Fogarty?

Fogarty balloon catheter—catheter with a balloon tip that can be inflated with saline; used for embolectomy/thrombectomy by insinuating the catheter with the balloon deflated past the embolus and then inflating the balloon and pulling the catheter out; the balloon brings the embolus with it

How many mm in diameter is a 12 French Fogarty catheter?

Simple; to get mm from French measurements divide the French number by pi or 3.14; thus a 12 French catheter is $12/3 = 4$ mm in diameter

What must you look for postop after reperfusion of the limb?	**COMPARTMENT SYNDROME,** hyperkalemia, renal failure due to myoglobinuria, MI
What is compartment syndrome?	The leg is separated into compartments by very unyielding fascia; **tissue swelling** due to reperfusion can cause an increase in the intracompartmental pressure, resulting in decreased capillary flow, ischemia, and myonecrosis; myonecrosis may occur after the intracompartment pressure reaches only 30 mm Hg
Signs/sx of a compartment syndrome?	Classic signs include pain, paralysis, paresthesias, and pallor; *pulses are present in most cases* because systolic pressure is quite higher than the minimal 30 mm Hg needed for the syndrome!
Can one have a pulse and a compartment syndrome?	**YES, YES,** AND **YES!**
Dx?	Hx/suspicion, measure compartment pressures
Rx compartment syndrome?	Treatment includes opening compartments via fasciotomies of all 4 compartments in the calf if pressures are >30–40 mm Hg or if patient is symptomatic

ABDOMINAL AORTIC ANEURYSMS

A.K.A.?	AAA or ''triple A''
What is it?	An abnormal dilation of the abdominal aorta forming an aneurysm
Common cause and location?	Nearly all are atherosclerotic (although the cause is thought to be multifactorial) (95%) and infrarenal (>95%); common underlying defect is vessel wall weakness secondary to loss of elastin/collagen
Incidence?	About 4% of white males (highest risk group), about 1 in 5 patients with PVD will have an AAA—thus r/o AAA in all your patients with PVD!
Risk factors? (5)	**Atherosclerosis,** hypertension, smoking, male gender, advancing age

Symptoms?	Most AAAs are *asymptomatic* and are discovered during routine abdominal exam by primary care physician; in the remainder, symptoms range from vague epigastric discomfort to back pain
Signs of rupture?	Classic triad of ruptured AAA: **abdominal pain, pulsatile abdominal mass, and hypotension;** pulsatile mass usually left of midline and above umbilicus. Severe back or flank pain and signs of blood loss suggests ruptured/leaking AAA; if a patient has the classic triad take the patient straight to the OR
Risk factors for rupture?	Recent rapid expansion, diameter, hypertension, COPD
What percentage rupture > 5 cm?	If untreated, about ⅓ of all AAA > 5 cm will rupture in 5 years!
Where does the aorta bifurcate?	At the level of the umbilicus; therefore when palpating for a AAA palpate above the umbilicus and below the xiphoid process
DDx?	Acute pancreatitis, dissecting aneurysm, mesenteric ischemia, MI, perforated ulcer, diverticulosis, renal colic
Diagnostic tests?	Use ULTRASOUND to follow AAA clinically; other tests involve contrast CT, and A-gram; A-gram will assess lumen patency and iliac/renal involvement (MRI is now being used with good results)
What is the limitation of A-gram?	AAAs often have large mural thrombi, which results in a falsely reduced diameter, as only the patent lumen is visualized
Signs of AAA on AXR?	Calcification in aneurysm wall seen best on lateral projection; A.K.A. egg-shell calcifications
Indications for surgical repair of AAA?	AAA over 5 cm, if patient does not have any overwhelming contraindications to surgery, and of course rupture of the AAA, rapid growth, symptoms
AAA grow by how much each year?	About 2–4 mm/year on average (larger AAAs grow faster than smaller AAAs)

Treatment?	Excision and prosthetic graft placement with rewrapping of the native aneurysm around the prosthetic graft after the thrombus is removed; when rupture is strongly suspected, start IV fluids, cross match blood, and **proceed to *immediate* laparotomy; no time for diagnostic test!**
Why wrap the graft in the native aorta?	**To reduce the incidence of enterograft fistula formation

OPERATIVE MORTALITY?

Elective?	Good; <4% operative mortality
Ruptured?	Poor; >50% operative mortality (if one includes those who die prior to reaching the hospital, the mortality of a ruptured AAA is about **90%**)
#1 cause of postoperative death in a patient undergoing elective AAA Rx?	**MYOCARDIAL INFARCTION****
Other etiologies of AAA?	Inflammatory (connective tissue diseases), mycotic (a misnomer as most due to bacteria **not** fungi) *salmonella*
Mean normal abdominal aortic diameter?	2 cm
Potential operative complications?	Atheroembolism, declamping hypotension, acute renal failure (especially if aneurysm involved the renal arteries), ureteral injury, myocardial ischemia arrhythmias, hemorrhage, stroke,
Why is colonic ischemia a concern in the repair of AAAs?	Often the IMA is sacrificed during surgery, which relies on collateral circulation to perfuse the left colon; if the collaterals are not adequate then the patient will have colonic ischemia
What are the signs of colonic ischemia?	Heme + stool, or BRBPR
What is the study of choice to diagnose colonic ischemia?	**Colonoscopy**
When do you see colonic ischemia postoperatively?	Usually in the first week postop

Long-term complication with upper/lower GI bleeding?	Aortoenteric fistula
Other postoperative complications?	Impotence (sympathetic plexus injury), retrograde ejaculation, aortovenous fistula (to IVC), graft infection, **anterior spinal syndrome**
What is the anterior spinal syndrome?	Classically: 1. Paraplegia 2. Loss of bladder/bowel control 3. Loss of pain/temperature sensation below level of involvement 4. **Sparing of proprioception Anterior spinal syndrome is due to spinal cord ischemia from cross clamping Ao (higher incidence with ruptured AAA)
What artery is involved in anterior spinal cord syndrome?	Artery of **Adamkiewicz**—supplies the anterior spinal cord
How do you treat a graft infection and aortoenteric fistula?	Perform an **extraanatomic bypass** with resection of the graft
What is an extraanatomic bypass graft?	Axillofemoral bypass graft—**graft not in a normal vascular path;** usually the graft goes from the axillary artery to the femoral artery and then from one femoral artery to the other (fem-fem bypass)

MESENTERIC ISCHEMIA

CHRONIC MESENTERIC ISCHEMIA _____

What is it?	Chronic intestinal ischemia due to long-term occlusion of the intestinal arteries; most commonly due to atherosclerosis; usually in 2 or more arteries due to the extensive collaterals
Sx/signs?	Weight loss, postprandial abdominal pain, +/− heme occult, +/− diarrhea
Dx?	Duplex ultrasound/Doppler, A-gram
Rx options?	Bypass, endarterectomy
What drug has been associated with intestinal ischemia?	Digitalis

ACUTE MESENTERIC ISCHEMIA _____

What is it?	Acute onset of intestinal ischemia
Causes?	Emboli from the heart, and thrombosis of long-standing atherosclerosis
Causes of emboli from heart?	MI, a. fib., cardiomyopathy, valve disease
Emboli go preferentially to which intestinal artery?	**SUPERIOR MESENTERIC ARTERY**
Signs/Sx of acute mesenteric ischemia?	Severe pain—classically "**pain out of proportion to physical exam,**" no peritoneal signs until necrosis, vomiting/diarrhea/hyperdefecation, +/− heme stools
Dx?	HISTORY/PE → A-gram; waste no time!
Rx emboli?	Fogarty catheter embolectomy, resect obviously necrotic intestine and leave marginal looking bowel until second-look laparotomy within 24 hours postop
Rx acute thrombosis?	Papaverine vasodilator via A-gram catheter until OR, then most would perform a supraceliac aorta graft to the involved intestinal artery; intestinal resection/second-look as needed

CEREBROVASCULAR DISEASE

What is it?	Usually emboli from a diseased carotid vessel or heart
Signs/Sx?	Amaurosis fugax, TIA, RIND, CVA

Define _____

Amaurosis fugax?	Temporary monocular blindness, "curtain coming down"; seen with microemboli to the retina; this is an example of a TIA
TIA?	Transient ischemic attack—focal neurologic deficit with resolution of all symptoms within 24 hours
RIND?	Reversible ischemic neurologic deficit = transient neurologic impairment (without any lasting sequelae) lasting 24–72 hours
CVA?	Cerebrovascular accident = stroke; neurologic deficit with permanent brain damage
Risk of CVA in patients with TIA?	About 10% a year! and about ⅓ will have a stroke in 5 years!

Noninvasive methods of evaluating carotid disease?	1. ****Carotid ultrasound/Doppler;** gives general location and degree of stenosis 2. **Oculoplethysmography:** measures indirectly the flow through the ophthalmic artery, the first branch off the carotid 3. **Supraorbital Doppler:** detects reversal of flow in the supraorbital arteries seen with occlusion of the internal carotid artery
Invasive method of evaluating carotid disease?	A-gram
Surgical Rx for carotid stenosis?	**CEA** = Carotid endarterectomy, the removal of the diseased intima and media of the carotid artery often performed with a shunt in place
Dreaded complications after a CEA?	STROKE! MI

SUBCLAVIAN STEAL SYNDROME

What is it?	Arm fatigue and vertebrobasilar insufficiency due to obstruction of the L subclavian artery proximal to the vertebral artery branch point; ipsilateral arm movement causes increased blood flow demand, which is met by retrograde flow from the vertebral artery, thereby "stealing" from the vertebrobasilar arteries
Sx?	UE claudication and those due to vertebrobasilar insufficiency: syncopal attacks, vertigo, confusion, dysarthria, blindness, or ataxia
Signs?	BP discrepancy with L UE < R UE blood pressure
Rx?	Surgical revision of the subclavian artery, but **rarely** indicated

RENAL ARTERY STENOSIS

What is it?	Stenosis of the renal artery resulting in decreased perfusion of the juxtaglomerular apparatus and subsequent activation of the aldosterone-renin-angiotensin system (i.e., hypertension due to renal artery stenosis)
Incidence?	• 10–15% of the U.S. population has HTN, and of these approx 4% have potentially correctable renovascular HTN • Also note that 30% of malignant HTN has a renovascular etiology

Etiology of the stenosis?

- ⅔ due to atherosclerosis (male > female)
- ⅓ due to fibromuscular dysplasia (female > male, average age 40 years, and 50% with bilateral disease)
- *Note:* another rare cause is hypoplasia of the renal artery

Risks?

Family hx, early onset of HTN, HTN that is refractory to medical Rx

Sx/signs?

Most are asymptomatic, but may have headache, *diastolic* **HTN,** flank bruits (present in 50%), and decreased renal function; *Note:* 7% of essential hypertensives also have flank bruits

Dx tests?

- *IVP:* 80% have delayed nephrogram phase (i.e., delayed filling of contrast)
- *Renal vein renin ratio* **(RVRR):** If sampling of renal vein renin levels shows ratio between the two kidneys ≥ 1.5, then diagnostic for a unilateral stenosis
- **Captopril provocation test:** Will show a drop in BP
- **Nuclear medicine renal scan:** Systemic renin levels may also be measured but are only increased in malignant HTN, as the increased intravascular volume dilutes the elevated renin level in most patients

Invasive nonsurgical Rx?

Percutaneous renal transluminal angioplasty (PRTA)
- Much better results with fibromuscular dysplasia, but also good for isolated short-segment atherosclerotic lesions away from the ostium of the renal artery
- With FM dysplasia: 85–100% success using PRTA and 5% restenosis rate
- With atherosclerosis: 40–90% success using PRTA and about ¼ restenosis
- Complications of PRTA: renal insufficiency, renal artery dissection and perforation, renal artery emboli, MI, and local complications at the femoral puncture site (pseudoaneurysm or massive bleeding)
Note: about 4% of patients undergoing PRTA require operative intervention

Surgical Rx?

Resection, bypass, vein/graft interposition, or endarterectomy

Medical Rx? Advisable Rx in a patient with generalized atherosclerotic disease and renal artery stenosis

SPLENIC ARTERY ANEURYSM

What is it? Aneurysm of the splenic artery

Causes? Women = medial dysplasia
Men = atherosclerosis

How diagnosed? Usually by abdominal pain → U/S, in OR after rupture, or incidentally by **egg-shell calcifications seen on AXR**

Risk factor for rupture? ****PREGNANCY**

POPLITEAL ARTERY ANEURYSM

What is it? Aneurysm of popliteal artery caused by atherosclerosis and rarely bacterial infection

Diagnosis? Most by physical exam → A-gram

Why examine the contralateral popliteal artery? **½ of all patients with a popliteal artery aneurysm have a popliteal artery aneurysm in the contralateral popliteal artery!**

Why examine the rest of the arterial tree (especially the abdominal Ao)? **¾ of all patients with popliteal aneurysms have additional aneurysms elsewhere!** with over ½ of these located in the abdominal Ao/iliacs!

SECTION *III*
Subspecialty Surgery

38
Pediatric Surgery

Motto of pediatric surgery?	"Children are NOT little adults!"
What is ECMO?	**E**xtra**c**orporeal **m**embrane **o**xygenation chronic cardiopulmonary bypass—for complete respiratory support
Maintance IV fluid for children?	D5 ¼ NS + 20 mEq KCl
Minimal urine output for children?	1–2 ml/kg/hr

NECK

Major differential diagnosis of a pediatric neck mass?	**Thyroglossal duct cyst (midline), branchial cleft cyst (lateral), lymphadenopathy, abscess, cystic hygroma, hemangioma, teratoma/dermoid cyst, thyroid nodule, lymphoma/leukemia, (also, parathyroid tumors, neuroblastoma, histiocytosis X, rhabdomyosarcoma, salivary gland tumors, neurofibroma)**

THYROGLOSSAL DUCT CYST _____

What is it?	Remnant of the diverticulum formed by the migration of thyroid tissue; normal development involves migration of thyroid tissue from foramen cecum at the base of the tongue through the hyoid bone to its final position around the tracheal cartilage
Average age at Dx?	Usually presents around 5 years of age
Method of Dx?	Ultrasound
Complications?	Enlargement, infection, and fistula formation between oropharynx or salivary gland; aberrant thyroid tissue may masquerade as a thyroglossal duct cyst, and if not cystic, deserves a thyroid scan
Anatomic location?	Almost always in **midline**

Rx?

Antibiotics if infected, then excision, which must include the midportion of the hyoid bone and the entire tract to foramen cecum (Sistrunk procedure)

BRANCHIAL CLEFT ANOMALIES

What is it?

Remnant of the primitive branchial clefts in which epithelium forms a sinus tract between the pharynx (2nd cleft), or the external auditory canal (1st cleft), and the skin of the anterior neck; if the sinus ends blindly a cyst may form

Common presentation?

Infection, because of communication between the pharynx and external ear canal

Anatomic position?

- 2nd cleft anomaly—**lateral to the midline** along the anterior border of the sternocleidomastoid, anywhere from the angle of the jaw to the clavicle
- 1st cleft anomaly—not as common as 2nd cleft anomalies; tend to be located higher under the mandible

Most common cleft remnant?

2nd; thus these are found most often laterally vs. thyroglossal cyst which are found centrally—key point**

Rx?

Abx if infection present, then surgical excision of cyst and tract once inflammation resolved

STRIDOR

What is it?

Harsh noise heard on breathing caused by obstruction of trachea or the larynx; often accounted for in the newborn by congenital malformations causing airway obstruction

Sx and Signs?

Dyspnea, cyanosis, difficulty with feedings

Differential Dx?

Laryngomalacia—#1 cause of stridor in the infant; results from inadequate development of supporting structures of the larynx, usually self-limited and Rx is expectant unless respiratory compromise present

Tracheobronchomalacia—similar to laryngomalacia, but involves entire trachea

Vascular rings and slings—abnormal development or placement of thoracic large vessels resulting in obstruction of trachea/bronchus

Sx of vascular rings?	Stridor, dyspnea on exertion, or dysphagia
Dx of vascular rings?	• Barium swallow revealing typical configuration of esophageal compression • Echo/arteriogram
Rx of vascular rings?	Surgical division of ring if the patient is symptomatic

CYSTIC HYGROMA

What is it?	Congenital abnormality of lymph sac resulting in lymphangioma
Anatomic location?	Occur in sites of primitive lymphatic lakes and can occur virtually anywhere in the body; most commonly in the floor of mouth, under jaw, in the neck, in the axilla, or in the thorax
Rx?	Early total surgical removal as they tend to enlarge; sclerosis may be needed if the lesion is unresectable
Complications?	Enlargement in critical regions such as floor of mouth or paratracheal region may cause obstruction of airway; also tend to insinuate onto major structures (although not malignant), making them difficult and hazardous to excise

CHEST

ESOPHAGEAL ATRESIA WITHOUT TRACHEOESOPHAGEAL FISTULA

What is it?	Blind-ending esophagus due to atresia
Signs?	Excessive oral secretions and inability to keep food down
Dx?	Inability to pass NG tube. Plain x-ray shows tube coiled in the upper esophagus and absence of gas in the abdomen
Primary Rx?	Suction blind pouch, IVFs, (gastrostomy to drain stomach if prolonged preop esophageal stretching is planned, to avoid aspiration of stomach contents)

Definitive Rx?   Surgical, often with preoperative stretching
                                      of blind pouch (other options include colonic
                                      or jejunal interposition graft or gastric tube
                                      formation if long esophageal gap)

ESOPHAGEAL ATRESIA WITH TRACHEOESOPHAGEAL FISTULA _____

What is it?   Esophageal atresia occurring with a fistula to
                                      the trachea, occurs in >90% of esophageal
                                      atresia

Incidence?   1 in 1500–3000 births

Types of Fistulas/Atresias _____

   Type A?   Type A—esophageal atresia without TE
                                      fistula (8%)

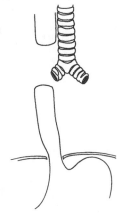

   Type B?   Type B—proximal esophageal atresia with
                                      proximal TE fistula (1%)

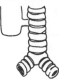

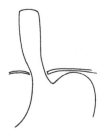

Type C?

Type C—proximal esophageal atresia with distal TE fistula (85%); ** **most common type**

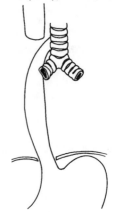

Type D?

Type D—proximal esophageal atresia with both proximal and distal TE fistulas (2%)

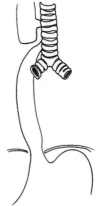

Type E?

Type E—''H-type'' TE fistula without esophageal atresia (4%)

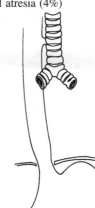

How do you remember which one is the most common type?	Simple, the most Common type = type C
Sx?	Excessive secretions caused by an accumulation of saliva (may not see with type E)
Signs?	Obvious respiratory compromise, aspiration pneumonia, postprandial regurgitation, gastric distention as air enters stomach directly from the trachea
Dx?	Failure to pass an NG tube (although this will not be seen with type E), plain film (avoid contrast because of high risk of aspiration) demonstrates tube coiled in the upper esophagus; distended stomach and small bowel causing elevated diaphragms also on plain film if connection airway (although this would not be seen with types A or B)
Initial Rx?	Directed toward minimizing complications from aspiration:

1. Suction blind pouch
2. Upright position of child
3. Prophylactic abx

Definitive Rx?	Surgical correction via a thoracotomy usually through right chest with division of fistula and end to end anastomosis if possible
Which type do you fix via a right neck incision?	"H-Type" (type E) is high in the thorax and can most often be approached via a right neck incision
Associated anomalies?	VACTERL cluster present in about 10%: Vertebral or Vascular, Anorectal, Cardiac, TE fistula, Esophageal atresia, Radial limb and Renal abnormalities, Lumbar & Limb.

CONGENITAL DIAPHRAGMATIC HERNIA

What is it?	Failure of complete formation of the diaphragm, leading to a defect through which abdominal organs herniate
Incidence?	1 in 2100 live births, males more commonly affected
Types of hernias?	Bochdalek and Morgagni

Position?	*Bochdalek*—posterolateral with L > R (think: ''Bochdalek = back to the left'')
	Morgagni—anterior parasternal hernia, relatively uncommon
Signs?	Respiratory distress as the presence of bowel in the thorax impedes lung development with lung hypoplasia in both lungs and pulmonary hypertension; dyspnea, tachypnea, retractions and cyanosis; at birth, swallowed air further distends the intestine, compressing the lung and causing a mediastinal shift, impeding venous return to the thorax and ventilation of the contralateral lung; may also auscultate bowel sounds in the chest
Rx?	NG tube, ET tube, stabilization, and if stable to OR for repair; if unstable to ECMO then to OR when deemed feasible

ABDOMEN

CONGENITAL PYLORIC STENOSIS

What is it?	Hypertrophy of the smooth muscle of the pylorus resulting in obstruction of outflow
Risks?	Family hx, firstborn males affected most commonly, decreased incidence in black population
Incidence?	1 in 500–750 births, M:F 4 to 1
Average age at onset?	Usually from 2 weeks after birth to about 2 months
Sx?	Increasing frequency of regurgitation leading to eventual *Nonbilious projectile vomiting,* wgt loss or lack of gain, decreasing frequency of stools
Signs?	Abdominal mass or ''olive'' in the epigastric region (85%), hypokalemic hypochloremic metabolic alkalosis, icterus (10%), visible gastric peristalsis, paradoxical aciduria, hematemesis (<10%)
Differential Dx?	Pylorospasm, milk allergy, increased ICP, hiatal hernia, GE reflux, adrenal insufficiency, uremia, malrotation, duodenal atresia, annular pancreas, duodenal web

Dx?

Most by hx and PE alone; ultrasound demonstrating elongated (>15mm) pyloric channel and thickened muscle wall (>3.5 mm); if US nondiagnostic, then barium swallow showing "string sign" or "double railroad track sign"

Initial Rx?

Hydration and correction of alkalosis with D10 NS plus 20–40 meq of KCl; *Note:* the infant's liver glycogen stores are very small, therefore use D10; Cl⁻ and hydration will correct the alkalosis

Definitive Rx?

Surgical via Fredet-Ramstedt pyloromyotomy (division of circular muscle fibers without entering the lumen/mucosa)

Postop complications?

Unrecognized incision through the duodenal mucosa, bleeding, wound infection, aspiration pneumonia

Postop feeding?

6–12 hr postop with sugar water and advance to full-strength formula over 24 hr

DUODENAL ATRESIA

What is it?

Complete obstruction or stenosis of duodenum caused by an ischemic insult during development, or failure of recanalization

Anatomic location?

85% distal to ampulla of Vater, 15% proximal to the ampulla of Vater (these present with nonbilious vomiting)

Signs?

Bilious vomiting (if distal to the ampulla), epigastric distention

Differential Dx?

Malrotation with Ladd's bands, annular pancreas

Dx?

Plain abdominal film revealing "double bubble"—with one air bubble in the stomach and the other in the duodenum

Rx?

Duodenoduodenostomy or duodenojejunostomy

Associated abnormalities?

50–70% have cardiac, renal, or other gastrointestinal defects; 30% have trisomy 21

JEJUNAL ATRESIA

What is it?	Obstruction due to atresia or stenosis resulting from a late mesenteric vascular accident caused by intrauterine volvulus, malrotation, internal hernia, intussusception, or strangulation in an abdominal wall defect
Classification?	Type I—mucosal web or diaphragm Type II—atretic cord between two blind ends with intact mesentery Type IIIa—complete separation with ''V-shaped'' mesentery defect ** **most common type** Type IIIb—''apple peel'' or ''Christmas tree'' deformity Type IV—instances of multiple atresia characterized by ''string of sausage'' appearance
Signs?	Bilious vomiting, abdominal distention, failure to pass meconium (not 100%), 3–4 air-fluid bubbles on plain films, jaundice (40%), microcolon due to disuse, hx of polyhydramnios (35%)
Primary Rx?	NG tube, fluid resuscitation
Definitive Rx?	Surgical resection of atretic loop with reanastomosis, with possible tapering of dilated proximal loop

ILEAL ATRESIA

What is it?	Similar process to jejunal atresia, but involving the ileum
Classification?	Same as jejunal atresia, type IIIa most common variant
Sx and signs?	Same as jejunal atresia
Definitive Rx?	Same as jejunal atresia
Complications?	Meconium peritonitis secondary to perforation in about 10%

MECONIUM ILEUS

What is it?	Intestinal obstruction due to solid meconium concretions

Incidence?	Occurs in about 15% of infants with cystic fibrosis, although almost all patients with meconium ileus have cystic fibrosis
Sx and signs?	Bilious vomiting, abdominal distention, failure to pass meconium, Neuhauser's sign—ground-glass appearance in the RLQ representing viscid meconium mixed with air
What is Neuhauser's sign?	A.K.A. "soap bubble" sign: on AXR, the meconium mixes with air and appears like ground glass
Dx?	Family hx of CF, plain abdominal films showing significant dilation of similar-sized bowel loops, but few if any air-fluid levels, BE may demonstrate "microcolon"
Rx?	Rx of choice is nonoperative clearance of meconium using Gastrografin enema, which is hypertonic and therefore draws fluid into the lumen, separating meconium pellets from bowel wall (50% success rate); if unsuccessful then enterotomy with intraoperative catheter irrigation

MECONIUM PERITONITIS

What is it?	A sign of intrauterine bowel perforation, as sterile meconium leads to an intense local inflammatory reaction with eventual formation of calcifications
Signs?	Calcifications on plain films

MECONIUM PLUG SYNDROME

What is it?	Colonic obstruction due to unknown factors that dehydrate meconium, forming a "plug"
Sx and Signs?	Abdominal distention and failure to pass meconium within first 24 hr of life; plain films demonstrate many loops of distended bowel and air-fluid levels
Rx?	Contrast enema is both diagnostic and therapeutic, demonstrates "microcolon" to point of dilated colon (usually in transverse colon) and reveals copious intraluminal material; *Note:* it may be confused with Hirschsprung's disease (5% of Hirschsprung's present in a similar manner)

Anorectal Malformations

What are they?	Malformations of the distal GI tract in the general categories of anal atresia, imperforate anus, and rectal atresia
Anal Atresia	Inappropriate ascent of proctoderm leading to a thin membrane covering the normal anal canal
Rx?	Puncture of the skin membrane, which is often protruding with meconium
Dx?	Physical examination

Anatomic variants?	• 90% have associated fistulous tract originating from the rectal segment
	• In males the fistulous tract is to the perineum (in low lesions) or the urethra (in high lesions)
	• In females there are more variants of fistulas
	    Rectoforchette fistula
	    Rectoperineal fistula
	    Rectovaginal fistula
	    Rectocloacal fistula

Rx?	Surgical correction → Pena posterior sagittal anoplasty
Associated anomalies?	Spinal dystrophic syndromes and other anomalies involving the GI tract, cardiovascular, genitourinary, and the musculoskeletal systems

Hirschsprung's Disease

Also known as?	Aganglionic megacolon
What is it?	Neurogenic form of intestinal obstruction in which absence of normal ganglion cells of the rectum and colon result in functional obstruction due to inadequate relaxation and peristalsis
Which plexuses are involved?	Myenteric (Auerbach's) and the submucosal (Meissner's) plexuses
Risks?	Family hx; 5% chance of having second child with affliction; 85% of cases are males
Anatomic location?	Aganglionosis begins at anorectal line and in 80% involves rectosigmoid (10% have involvement to splenic flexure and 10% have involvement of entire colon)

Sx and Signs?	Abdominal distention and bilious vomiting; > 95% present with failure to pass meconium in the first 24 hr; can also present later with constipation, diarrhea, and decreased growth
Differential Dx?	Hypothyroidism, meconium plug syndrome, sepsis with adynamic ileus, colonic neuronal dysplasia
Dx?	Unprepared barium enema reveals constricted aganglionic segment with dilated proximal segment, but this picture may not develop for 3–6 weeks; BE will also demonstrate retention of barium for 24–48 hr, (normal evacuation = 10–18 hr) *Rectal biopsy* for definitive Dx, Submucosal suction Bx adequate in 90% of cases; otherwise do full thickness Bx to evaluate Auerbach's plexus
Rx?	In neonates, a colostomy proximal to the transition zone prior to correction, to allow for pelvic growth and dilated bowel to return to normal size Definitive correction via either Duhamel, Swenson, or Soave pullthrough procedures
Swenson?	**Swenson**—generally, a primary anastomosis between anal canal and healthy bowel (rectum removed)
Duhamel?	**Duhamel**—the anterior, aganglionic region of the rectum is preserved and anastomosed to a posterior portion of healthy bowel; a functional rectal pouch is thereby created; (Think: duha = dual barrels side by side)
Soave?	**Soave**—A.K.A. endorectal pullthrough; this procedure involves bringing proximal normal colon through the aganglionic rectum, which has been stripped of its mucosa but otherwise present; (think: *soave* = *save* the rectum)
Prognosis?	Overall survival >90%; >96% are continent and postoperative sx improve with age
Associations?	3–5% have trisomy 21

MALROTATION AND MIDGUT VOLVULUS

What is it?	Failure of the normal bowel rotation, with resultant abnormal intestinal attachments and anatomic positions

Where is the cecum?	With malrotation the cecum ends up in the RUQ
What are Ladd's bands?	Fibrous bands that extend from the abnormally placed cecum in the RUQ, often crossing over the duodenum and causing obstruction
Age at onset?	⅓ present in the first wk of life 85% recognized by one year
Usual presentation?	Sudden onset of bilious vomiting—BILIOUS VOMITING IN INFANT IS MALROTATION UNTIL PROVEN OTHERWISE!
Dx?	BE or upper GI series with follow-through, the BE showing abnormal position of the cecum in the upper abdomen
Complications?	Volvulus with midgut infarction leading to death or necessitating massive enterectomy; *rapid Dx is essential!*
Rx?	IV abx and fluid rescusitation with LR, followed by emergent laparotomy with reduction of volvulus
	Appendectomy is also performed to avoid possible difficulty with Dx in future; second-look laparotomy if necessary in 24–36 hr to determine if remaining bowel is viable
How does one reduce the volvulus?	Rotate the bowel in a **counterclockwise** direction
After reduction where is the cecum?	In the LLQ
Mortality?	15–25% mortality for midgut volvulus
Associated abnormalities?	Congenital diaphragmatic hernias, abdominal wall defects, and duodenal atresia

OMPHALOCELE

What is it?	Defect of the umbilical ring; extruded viscera are **covered** by sac
What comprises the "sac"?	Peritoneum and amnion
Incidence?	About 1 in 5000 births

Dx?	Prenatal ultrasound
Rx?	1. NG tube for decompression 2. IVFs 3. Prophylactic abx 4. Surgical repair of defect
Small defect (<2 cm)?	Closure of abdominal wall
Medium defect?	Remove outer membrane and place silicone patch to form "silo" to temporarily house abdominal contents; the silo is then slowly decreased in size over 4–7 days, as the abdomen accommodates the viscera; then the defect is closed
Large defects (>10 cm)?	Most are treated with Betadine spray or Silvadene over the defect, allowing an eschar to form, which epithelializes over time, allowing opportunity for future repair months to years later
Associated abnormalities?	50% of cases occur with often severe abnormalities of GI tract, cardiovascular system, genitourinary tract, musculoskeletal system, CNS, and chromosomes

GASTROSCHISIS

What is it?	Defect of the abdominal wall; extruded viscera not covered by sac
Where is the defect?	**Lateral to umbilicus (R > L).**
Complications?	Thick edematous peritoneum due to exposure to amnionic fluid; nonrotation of gut; other complications include hypothermia, hypovolemia due to third-spacing, sepsis, and metabolic acidosis due to hypovolemia and poor perfusion
Dx?	Prenatal ultrasound
Rx?	*Primary*—NG tube decompression, IVFs (D10 LR), and IV abx *Definitive*—Surgical reduction of viscera and abdominal closure; may require staged closure with silo
What is a "SILO"?	Silastic silo is a temporary housing for external abdominal contents; silo is slowly tightened over time; *Note:* a prolonged postop adynamic ileus requiring TPN for adequate caloric support may be present

Prognosis?	>90% survival
Associated anomalies?	Unlike omphalocele, relatively uncommon, except for intestinal atresia which occurs in 10–15%
Major differences from omphalocele?	No coverings Uncommon associated abnormalities

APPENDICITIS

What is it?	Obstruction of the appendiceal lumen producing a closed loop with resultant inflammation that can lead to necrosis and perforation
Presentation?	Onset of referred or periumbilical pain followed by anorexia, nausea and vomiting; *Note:* unlike gastroenteritis *pain precedes vomiting;* pain then migrates to the RLQ where it becomes more intense and localized due to local peritoneal irritation; also note the presentation may vary depending on the anatomical location of the appendix *If the patient is hungry and can eat—seriously question the diagnosis of appendicitis
Dx?	History and physical exam
Signs and Sx?	Signs of peritoneal irritation may be present—guarding, muscle spasm, rebound tenderness, obturator and psoas signs, low-grade fever rising to high grade if perforation occurs
Differential Dx?	Intussusception, volvulus, Meckel's diverticulum, Crohn's disease, ovarian torsion, cyst, tumor, perforated ulcer, pancreatitis, PID, ruptured ectopic pregnancy, mesenteric lymphadenitis
Labs?	Increased WBC (> 10,000 per mm^3 in >90% of cases) UA to rule out pyelonephritis or renal calculus **Mild hematuria and pyuria are *very* common in appendicitis with pelvic inflammation

What is the "hamburger" sign?	Ask patients with suspected appendicitis if they would like a hamburger or their favorite food—if they can really eat, seriously question the diagnosis
Radiographic studies?	CXR to r/o RML or RLL pneumonia, abdominal films usually nonspecific, but calcified fecalith present in 5%
Rx?	If not perforated, prompt appy + cefoxitin avoid perforation; if perforated, triple abx, fluid rescusitation, and prompt appendectomy; all pus is drained and cultures obtained with postop abx continued for 5–7 days
If one finds a normal appendix upon exploration, what must one exam/rule out?	Meckel's diverticulum, Crohn's disease, intussusception
Risk of perforation?	25% after 24 hr from onset of sx 50% by 36 hr 75% by 48 hr

INTUSSUSCEPTION

What is it?	Obstruction caused by bowel telescoping into the lumen of adjacent distal bowel; may result when a "leadpoint" is carried downstream by peristalsis
Age at presentation?	Disease of infancy; 60% present from 4–12 months, 80% by age 2 years
Most common site?	Terminal ileum involving ileocecal valve and into the ascending colon
Most common cause?	Hypertrophic Peyer's patches which act as lead points; many patients have prior viral illness
Signs and Sx?	Alternating lethargy and irritability (colic), bilious vomiting, "currant jelly" stools, RLQ mass on plain abdominal film, empty RLQ on palpation (Dance's sign)
What is the intussuscipiens?	The recipient segment of bowel (think: "recipiens" = intussus"cipiens")
What is the intussusceptum?	The leading point or bowel that enters the intussuscipiens

Classic question: How do you spell intussusception????	Intussusception—2 "s" followed by 1 "s" or 2,1 (not 1,2!)
Rx?	Air or barium enema; 85% reduce with hydrostatic pressure; if unsuccessful, then laparotomy and reduction by "milking" the ileum from the colon; *Note:* most surgeons also perform appendectomy at that time; if these fail, then resection with end to end
Causes of intussusception in older populations?	Meckel's diverticulum, polyps, and tumors, which all act as lead points

Meckel's Diverticulum

What is it?	Remnant of the omphalomesenteric duct/ vitelline duct, which connects the yolk sac with the primitive midgut in the embryo
Usual location?	45–90 cm proximal to the ileocecal valve on the antimesenteric border of the bowel
Major differential diagnosis?	**APPENDICITIS**
Is it a true diverticulum?	Yes, all layers of the intestine are found in the wall
Incidence?	Up to 3% of the population at autopsy, but >90% of these are asymptomatic
Sex ratio?	3× more common in males
Age at onset of Sx?	Most frequently in the first 2 years of life, but can occur at any age
Complications?	*Intestinal hemorrhage* (painless)—50% Accounts for half of all lower GI bleeding in patients < 2 years; bleeding due to ectopic gastric mucosa secreting acid → ulcer → bleeding *Intestinal obstruction*—25% Most common complication in adults; includes volvulus and intussusception *Inflammation* (+/− perforation)—20%
Heterotopic tissue?	Present in >50% of cases; usually (85%) is gastric mucosa, but duodenal, pancreatic, and colonic mucosa have been described
What other pediatric disease entity can also present with GI bleeding secondary to ectopic gastric mucosa?	Enteric duplications

Most common cause of lower GI bleeding in children?	Meckel's diverticulum with ectopic gastric mucosa
Rule of "2s"?	• 2% are symptomatic • Found about 2 feet from the ileocecal valve • Found in 2% of the population
What is a Meckel's scan?	Scan for ectopic gastric mucosa in Meckel's diverticulum; uses technetium pertechnetate IV, which is preferentially taken up by gastric mucosa

NECROTIZING ENTEROCOLITIS

A.K.A.?	NEC
What is it?	Necrosis of intestinal mucosa often with bleeding; may progress to transmural intestinal necrosis, shock/sepsis, and death
Predisposing conditions?	*Stress:* shock, hypoxia, RDS, apneic episodes, sepsis, exchange transfusions, PDA and cyanotic heart disease, hyperosmolar feedings, polycythemia, indomethacin
Pathophysiologic mechanism?	Probable splanchnic vasoconstriction with decreased perfusion, mucosal injury and probable bacterial invasion
Claim to infamy?	**Most common cause of emergent laparotomy in the neonate**
Sx and signs?	Abdominal distention, vomiting, heme + or gross rectal bleeding, fever or hypothermia, jaundice, abdominal wall erythema (consistent with perforation and abscess formation)
Radiographic findings?	Fixed, dilated intestinal loops, pneumatosis intestinalis (air in the bowel wall), free air, and portal vein air (sign of advanced disease)
Lab findings?	Low Hct, Low glucose, low platelets
Rx?	¾ managed medically: 1. Cessation of feedings 2. OG tube 3. IVFs 4. IV abx 5. Ventilator support as needed

Surgical indications?	Free air in abdomen revealing perforation and positive peritoneal tap revealing transmural bowel necrosis
Indications for peritoneal tap?	Severe thrombocytopenia, distended abdomen, abdominal wall erythema, unexplained clinical downturn
Complications?	Occur commonly and include further bowel necrosis, Gram-negative sepsis, DIC, wound infection, cholestasis, short bowel syndrome, and strictures; long term: small bowel obstruction
Prognosis?	>80% survive overall

BILIARY TRACT

BILIARY ATRESIA

What is it?	Obliteration of extrahepatic biliary tree
Incidence?	1 in 16000 births
Signs and Sx?	Persistent jaundice (nl physiologic jaundice resolves in <2 weeks), hepatomegaly, splenomegaly, ascites and other signs of portal hypertension, acholic stools, biliuria
Labs?	Mixed jaundice always present (i.e., both direct and indirect bilirubin increased), elevated serum alkaline phosphatase
Differential Dx?	Neonatal hepatitis (TORCH); biliary hypoplasia
Dx?	1. US to r/o choledochal cyst and to examine extrahepatic bile ducts and gallbladder 2. IDA scan—shows no excretion into GI tract (with phenobarb preparation) 3. Operative cholangiogram and liver bx
Rx?	Early laparotomy by 2 months of age with a modified form of the Kasai hepatoportoenterostomy
How does a Kasai work?	The anastomosis of the porta hepatis and the small bowel allows drainage of bile via many microscopic bile ducts in the fibrous structure of the porta hepatis
What if the Kasai fails?	Revise or liver transplantation

Postop complications?   Cholangitis (manifested as decreased bile secretion, fever, leukocytosis, and recurrence of jaundice), progressive cirrhosis (manifested as portal hypertension with bleeding varices, ascites, hypoalbuminemia, hypothrombinemia, and fat-soluble vitamin K, A, D, E deficiencies

Associated abnormalities?   25–30% have other anomalies including annular pancreas, duodenal atresia, malrotation, polysplenic syndrome, situs inversus, and preduodenal portal vein; 15% have congenital heart defects

CHOLEDOCHAL CYST

What is it?   Cystic enlargement of the bile ducts; most commonly arises in the extrahepatic ducts but can also arise in intrahepatic ducts

Presentation?   50% present with intermittent jaundice, RUQ mass, and abdominal pain; may also present with pancreatitis

Complications?   Cholelithiasis, cirrhosis, carcinoma, and portal HTN

Anatomic variants?   I. Dilation of common hepatic and common bile duct, with cystic duct entering the cyst; most common type

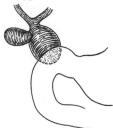

Type I

II. Lateral saccular cystic dilation

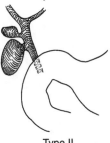

Type II

III. Choledochocele represented by an intraduodenal cyst

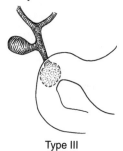

Type III

IV. Multiple extrahepatic cysts, intrahepatic cysts, or both

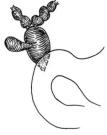

Type IV

V. Single or multiple intrahepatic cysts

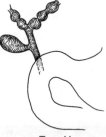

Type V

Dx?   Ultrasound

Rx?   Operative cholangiogram to clarify
                           pathologic process and delineate the
                           pancreatic duct, followed by complete
                           resection of the cyst and a Roux-en-Y
                           hepatojejunostomy

These patients have increased risk of what?	Cholangiocarcinoma often arises in cyst, thus Rx by the complete prophylactic resection of the cyst

CHOLELITHIASIS _____

What is it?	The formation of gallstones
Common causes in children?	*Note:* the etiology differs somewhat from adults; most common cause still cholesterol stones, but increased percentage of pigmented stones due to hemolytic disorders
Differential Dx?	Hereditary spherocytosis, thalassemia, pyruvate kinase deficiency, Sickle cell disease, cystic fibrosis, long-term parenteral nutrition, idiopathic
Risks?	Use of oral contraceptives, teenage pregnancy, + family hx
Dx?	Ultrasound and ERCP when indicated
Rx?	Cholecystectomy

TUMORS

WILMS' TUMOR _____

What is it?	Embryonal tumor of renal origin
Incidence?	500 new cases in the U.S. per year
Average age at Dx?	1–4 yr of age
Sx?	Usually asymptomatic except for abdominal mass; 20% present with minimal blunt trauma to mass
Signs?	Abdominal mass (most do not cross the midline); hematuria (10–15%); hypertension in 20% and related to compression of juxtaglomerular apparatus
Dx?	Physical exam, abdominal CT with IV contrast to evaluate collecting system, CXR to r/o lung metastases

Staging _____

Stage I?	Limited to kidney and completely resected
Stage II?	Extends beyond kidney, but completely resected; capsule invasion and perirenal tissues may be involved

Stage III?	Residual nonhematogenous tumor confined to abdomen
Stage IV?	Hematogenous metastases (lung, distal lymph nodes, and brain)
Stage V?	Bilateral renal involvement
Best indicator of survival?	Histological subtype of tumor; 85% have favorable histology (FH); 15% have unfavorable histology (UH); overall survival for FH is 90% for all stages
Rx?	Radical resection of affected kidney with evaluation for staging, followed by chemotherapy/radiation
Associated abnormalities?	Aniridia, hemihypertrophy, Beckwith-Wiedemann syndrome, neurofibromatosis, and horseshoe kidney
What is the Beckwith-Wiedemann syndrome?	**Syndrome of** 1. Exomphalos (umbilical hernia) 2. Macroglossia (big tongue) 3. Gigantism 4. Visceromegaly (big organs)

NEUROBLASTOMA

What is it?	Embryonal tumor of neural crest origin
Anatomic locations?	Neck—3% Posterior mediastinum—20% Pelvis—3% Paraaortic paraspinal ganglia—25% *Adrenal medulla—50%
Incidence?	1 in 7000–10,000 live births; most common solid malignant tumor of infancy
Average age at Dx?	50% by 2 yr 90% by 8 yr
Sx?	Vary by tumor location—anemia, failure to thrive, wgt loss, and poor nutritional status with advanced disease
Signs?	Asymptomatic abdominal mass (palpable in 50%), respiratory distress (mediastinal tumors), Horner's syndrome (upper chest or neck tumors), proptosis (with orbital metastases), subcutaneous tumor nodules, HTN (20–35%)

Dx?	Physical exam, 24-hr urine to measure VMA, HVA, and metanephrines (elevated in >85%), plain radiographs (may show calcifications), CXR, CT, and bone marrow bx to r/o metastases, ferritin, neuron-specific enolase, N-*myc* oncogene, DNA ploidy
Anatomy of tumor in neuroblastoma vs. Wilms'?	Neuroblastoma may cross midline, but Wilms' does so only rarely
Rx?	Depends on staging
Stage I?	(5% of cases); tumor confined to organ of origin Rx—complete excision Survival—approx. 100%
Stage II?	(25% of cases); tumor extends beyond organ of origin, but not across midline Rx—excision +/− chemo Survival—approx. 80%
Stage III?	(20% of cases); tumor extends across midline Rx—excision if possible, otherwise chemo to shrink tumor with second-look resection Survival—approx. 30%
Stage IV?	(50% of cases); metastatic disease Rx—Multiple drug chemo with resection, or local irradiation for residual nonresectable tumor, or total body irradiation plus Melphalan therapy and rescue with autologous bone marrow transplant Survival—approx 12%
Stage IVS?	Localized primary tumor not crossing the midline, but with remote disease confined to the liver, subcutaneous tissues, and bone marrow Rx controversial Survival >80%! note survival compared with stage IV! *Note:* these tumors are basically stage I or II with mets to liver, subQ tissue, or bone marrow; most of these patients if under 1 year of age have a spontaneous cure!
Key indicators of survival?	Age and stage, with $\frac{3}{4}$ of children <1 yr surviving; $\frac{1}{3}$ survival in children >1 yr of age
Laboratory prognostigators?	Aneuploidy is favorable! the lower the number of N-*myc* oncogene copies the better the prognosis

Oncogene associated with neuroblastoma?	N-*myc* oncogene

RHABDOMYOSARCOMA

What is it?	Highly malignant striated muscle sarcoma
Claim to infamy?	Most common sarcoma in children
Dx?	Tissue Bx, CT, MRI
Sx?	Mass
Rx?	Depends on location, stage, and tumor histology; may involve excision, chemotherapy, and radiation therapy
Overall survival?	70% at 3 years 55% at 5 years

HEPATOBLASTOMA

What is it?	Malignant tumor of the liver (derived from embryonic liver cells)
Average age at Dx?	Presents in first 3 years of life
Dx?	• Physical exam—abdominal distention; RUQ mass that moves with respiration • Elevated serum α-fetoprotein and ferritin (can be used as tumor markers) • CT scan of the abdomen, which often predicts resectability
Rx?	Resection by lobectomy or trisegmentectomy is Rx of choice; large tumors may require preop chemotherapy and subsequent hepatic resection, transplant

Staging
  I?
  II?
  III?
  IV?
	
	Completely resected
	Resected with microscopic residual disease
	Unresected tumor or gross residual disease
	Metastatic disease (usually to lung)

Overall survival?	50%
Major difference in age presentation between hepatoma and hepatoblastoma?	Hepatoblastoma presents < 3 yr of age; hepatoma > 3 yr and adolescents

OTHER PEDIATRIC SURGERY QUESTIONS

What is bilious vomiting in an infant?	MALROTATION UNTIL PROVEN OTHERWISE! (about 90% of patients with malrotation present before their first year of life)
What does TORCHES stand for?	Nonbacterial fetal and neonatal infx: **T**oxoplasmosis, **R**ubella, **C**ytomegalovirus (CMV), **H**erpes, **S**yphilis.
Common pediatric sedative?	Chloral hydrate
Contraindication to circumcision?	Hypospadias, etc., as the foreskin might be needed for future repair of the abnormality!
When to repair an umbilical hernia?	If older than at least 2 years age and if hernia defect is more than 1.5 cm in diameter; otherwise observe, as most close spontaneously
Cancer risk in the cryptorchid testicle?	$> 10 \times$ normal testicular cancer rate
When to perform orchidopexy?	All patients with undescended testicle undergo orchidopexy after 1 year of life
Signs of child abuse?	Cigarette burns, rope burns, scald to posterior thighs and buttocks, multiple fractures/old fractures, genital trauma, delay in accessing health care system
Rx for child abuse?	ADMIT THE PATIENT to the hospital
How does one treat the vast majority of splenic injuries in children?	6 weeks of bedrest
What is the role of DPL in children?	Much less a role than with adults, as most centers either go to the O.R. or the CT scanner to evaluate the abdomen
Common simulator of peritoneal signs in the blunt pediatric trauma victim?	Gastric distention—place an NGT
What is Dance's sign?	Empty RLQ in patients with ileocecal intussusception
Rx for hemangioma?	Observe, as most regress spontaneously

Indications for operation in hemangiomas?

Severe thrombocytopenia, congestive heart failure, functional impairment (vision, breathing)

Rx options for hemangiomas?

Steroids, radiation, surgical resection, angiographic embolization

Most common benign liver tumor in children?

Hemangioma

What is Eagle-Barret's syndrome?

A.K.A. prune belly; congenital inadequate abdominal musculature (very lax and thin)

Most common cancers in children?

#1 Leukemia
#2 CNS tumors
#3 Lymphomas

Most common solid neoplasm in infants?

Neuroblastoma

Most common solid tumor in children?

CNS tumors

What syndrome must you consider in the patient with abdominal pain, hematuria, hx of joint pain and a purpuric rash?

Henoch-Schonlein syndrome; also may have melena (50%) or at least guaiac + stools in about 75%

How do you spell guaiac?

Don't cheat—GUAIAC

What is Apley's law?

The farther a chronically recurrent abdominal pain is from the umbilicus, the greater the likelihood of an organic cause for the pain

Most common cause of SBO in children?

HERNIAS**

What is a patent urachus?

Persistence of the urachus, a communication between the bladder and the umbilicus; presents with urine out the umbilicus and recurrent UTIs

Risk after peanut aspiration?

Lipoid pneumonia

What is Ballance's sign?

Tender mass felt in LUQ in patients with splenic injury

What is Chiladidee's sign?

Loop of bowel over liver simulating free air under diaphragm on AXR

What is an annular pancreas?   Congenital pancreatic abnormality with complete encirclement of the duodenum by the pancreas

Sx of annular pancreas?   Duodenal obstruction

Rx annular pancreas?   Duoduodenostomy bypass of obstruction

39
Plastic Surgery

WOUND HEALING

Name 3 stages of wound healing

1. Lag or **inflammatory phase**
2. Fibroblastic or **proliferative phase**—collagen content and wound site strength increase
3. Maturation or **remodeling phase**—improvement in wound appearance, lasts several years

Wounds with skin loss require the same phases of healing and what 2 additional mechanisms?

1. Epithelialization
2. Wound contraction

EPITHELIALIZATION _____

What degree of bacterial contamination prevents epithelialization?

>100,000 organisms/gm tissue (10^5)

What structures does the epithelium grow in from in superficial burns/wounds?

Sweat glands and hair follicles

In full-thickness burns?

From wound margins, since no sweat glands or hair remains; this epithelium has no underlying dermis and is susceptible to injury

What malignant ulcer is associated with a long-standing scar/burn?

Marjolin's ulcer (A.K.A. burn scar carcinoma)

What is Fournier's gangrene?

Necrotizing cellulitis and fascitis of the *perineum* **of diabetics;** often leaves a massive wound after debridement

WOUND CONTRACTION _____

What are myofibroblasts?

Specialized fibroblasts that behave like smooth muscle cells to pull the wound edges together following granulation

How do we slow this contraction?	Split thickness skin grafts (STSG)
How do we stop it?	Full-thickness skin grafts (FTSG)
Which contracts more, an STSG or FTSG?	An STSG contracts up to 41% in surface area, while a FTSG contracts little if any at all
What is granulation tissue?	Within 4–6 days after an open wound, development of capillary beds and fibroblasts provides a healthy base for epithelial growth from wound edges; this tissue also resists bacterial infection

Name 3 local factors that impair wound healing

1. Low oxygen tension; tight sutures and dressings; IDDM; elderly with small vessel disease; radiation (obliterates small vessels); fibrosis
2. Hematoma or seroma—impairs apposition of wound edges and provides excellent culture medium for bacteria
3. Surgical technique—collagen and collagen lysis are at war during wound healing; infection, steroids, and poorly placed sutures will favor collagen lysis and will delay restoration of the strength of the wound

Name 4 general factors delaying wound healing

1. **Nutrition**—e.g., vitamin C deficiency causes decreased hydroxylation of proline and lysine, so new collagen formation is impaired; zinc is needed for burns, trauma, and septic patients
2. **Steroids**—especially in the first 4 days following injury, as they inhibit the normal resistance to infection and wound healing
3. **Sepsis**—probably impairs the utilization of amino acids used to form collagen
4. **Cytotoxic drugs**—suppression of fibroblast replication and collagen synthesis

What can help wound healing in patients on steroids?	Vitamin A is thought to counteract the deleterious effect of steroids on wound healing
When does a wound gain > 80% of its maximal tensile strength?	After approx. 6 weeks

DEFINE _____

Laceration?	*Torn/mangled/cut wound*
Abrasion?	Superficial skin removal
Contusions?	Bruise without break in skin
Keloid?	Hypertrophic scar

Skin Prep

Is it a good idea to shave the skin prior to surgery?

No; it increases the risk of infection by increasing the bacterial levels tenfold or more

Do anesthetic prep solutions help in wound healing?

No; they may worsen the environment for healing. Those containing ETOH or H_2O_2 are lethal to healthy cells as well as to bacteria

Components of a good prep?

Don't put it in the wound if you wouldn't put it in your eye; a simple balanced salt solution is a good prep and irrigant; don't forget adequate anesthesia; even when dirt is visible in the wound, infiltrate first, then irrigate and debride

Why not clean lacerations with Betadine?

Betadine is harmful to and inhibits normal healthy tissue

SKIN GRAFTS

What is a split-thickness skin graft?

Includes the epidermis and a variable amount of the dermis

How thick is it?

$^{12}/_{1000}$ to $^{18}/_{1000}$ inch

What is a full-thickness skin graft?

It involves the entire epidermis and dermis

Prerequisites for skin to take?

The bed must be vascularized—a graft graft to a bone or tendon will not take; bacteria < 100,000; shearing motion and fluid beneath the graft must be minimized

What is "tie-over bolus dressing"?

In an area that does not lend itself to circumferential wrapping, a tie-over dressing provides continuous compression to skin grafts in concave wounds; the skin graft is fixed to the recipient site with long sutures and then is covered with xeroform; a bolus of cotton is then applied and the sutures on opposite side are pulled together to hold the packing in place

FLAPS

Random flap—where does it get its blood supply?
From the dermal-subdermal plexus

Axial flap ... ?
It is vascularized by direct cutaneous arteries

Name some axial flaps and their arterial supply
Forehead flap—superficial temporal a.; often used for intraoral lesions
Deltopectoral flap—2nd, 3rd, & 4th anterior perforators of the internal mammary a.; often used for head and neck wounds
Groin flap—superficial circumflex iliac a.; allows coverage of hand and forearm wounds.

What is a "free flap"?
Flap separated from all vascular supply requires anastomosis

What is a TRAM flap?
Transverse **r**ectus **a**bdominis **m**yocutaneous flap

HANDS

Where is "no man's land"?
Flexor hand lacerations anywhere from the middle of the middle phalanx to the distal palmer crease need to be repaired by a hand expert

What hand laceration should be left unsutured?
Lacerations due to human bites

Most effective way to clean a laceration?
H_2O irrigation

Should you ever use a clamp to stop a laceration bleeder?
No, use pressure and then tourniquet for definitive repair if bleeding does not cease, as **nerves run with blood vessels!**

What is a FELON?
Infection in tip of finger pad (think of felon = fingerprints = infection in pad); Rx by drainage.

What is a PARONCHIA?
Infection on side of finger nail; Rx by drainage.

What is tenosynovitis?
Tendon sheath infection

What are Kanavel's signs?
Kanavel's 4 signs of tenosynovitis:
1. Affected finger held in slight **flexion**
2. **Pain** over volar aspect of affected finger tendon upon **palpation**
3. **Swelling** of affected finger
4. **Pain on passive extension** of affected finger

How does one Rx a human hand bite?	Debride/irrigate/antibiotics
What is the most common hand/wrist tumor?	**Ganglion cyst**
What is a "boxer's fracture"?	Fracture of 4th or 5th metacarpal

DEFINE

Syndactyly	Webbed fingers
Polydactyly	Extra fingers
Mammoplasty	Breast surgery (reduction/augmentation)
Facelift	Removal of excess facial skin via hairline/chin/ear incisions
Blepharoplasty	Eyelid surgery—removing excess skin/fat
Rhinoplasty	Nose surgery, after trauma or cosmetic
What are Langer's lines?	The natural direction/alignment of connective tissue in the dermis (e.g., transverse lines across abdomen); incisions perpendicular to Langer's lines result in larger scars than incision parallel to the lines

40
Otolaryngology—Head and Neck Surgery

EAR

Otitis Externa (Swimmer's Ear)

What is it?

Generalized infection involving the external ear canal and often the tympanic membrane

Usual cause?

Prolonged water exposure + damaged squamous epithelium of the ear canal (i.e., swimming, hearing aid use)

Typical pathogens?

Most frequently ***Pseudomonas,*** may be *Proteus, Staphylococcus,* occasionally fungi (*Aspergillus, Candida*), or virus (herpes zoster or herpes simplex)

Signs/Sx?

Ear pain (otalgia), external ear and/or ear canal swelling, erythema, pain on manipulation of the auricle, debris in canal

Treatment?

Most importantly, keep ear dry. Mild infections respond to cleaning and dilute acetic acid drops. Most infections require complete removal of all debris and topical abx ± hydrocortisone (antiinflammatory); consider antifungal drops for otomycosis

Malignant Otitis Externa

What is it?

Fulminant **bacterial** otitis externa

Who is affected?

Most common scenario: an elderly, poorly controlled diabetic (other forms of immunosuppression do not appear to predispose toward MOE)

Causative organisms?

Usually ***Pseudomonas aeruginosa***

Classic feature?

A nub of granulation tissue on the floor of the external ear canal at the bony-cartilaginous junction.

Other Signs/Sx?	Severe ear pain, excessive purulent discharge, and usually exposed bone
Complications?	Invasion of surrounding structures to produce a cellulitis, osteomyelitis of temporal bone, mastoiditis; later a facial nerve palsy, meningitis, or brain abscess
Treatment?	Control of patient's diabetes, meticulous local care with extensive debridement, hospitalization and IV abx (anti-*Pseudomonas;* usu. an aminoglycoside + a penicillin)

TUMORS OF THE EXTERNAL EAR

Most common types?	Squamous cell is most common; occ. basal cell carcinoma or melanoma
Usually arise from?	The auricle, but occasionally arise from external canal
Risk factor?	Excessive sun exposure

Treatment

Cancers of the auricle?	Usually treated by wedge excision
Extension to the canal?	May require excision of the external ear canal, or partial temporal bone excision
Middle ear involvement?	Best treated by en bloc temporal bone resection

TYMPANIC MEMBRANE (TM) PERFORATION

Etiology?	Usually the result of trauma (direct or indirect) or secondary to middle ear infection; often occurs secondary to slap to the side of the head (compression injury)
Symptoms?	Pain, conductive hearing loss, tinnitus
Signs?	Bleeding from ear, clot in meatus, visible tear in TM
Treatment?	Keep dry; use systemic abx if evidence of infection or contamination
Prognosis?	Most (90%) heal spontaneously, though larger perfs may require surgery

CHOLESTEATOMA _____

What is it?	An epidermal inclusion cyst of the middle ear or mastoid, containing desquamated keratin debris; may be acquired or congenital
Causes?	Negative middle ear pressure (primary acquired; typically in attic) or direct growth of epithelium through a TM perforation (secondary acquired)
Often associated with?	Chronic middle ear infection
Usual history?	Chronic ear infection with chronic, malodorous drainage
Appearance?	Grayish-white, shiny keratinous mass behind or involving the TM; often described as a ''pearly'' lesion
Associated problems?	Ossicular erosion, producing conductive hearing loss; also: local invasion resulting in vertigo/sensorineural hearing loss facial paresis/paralysis CNS dysfunction
Treatment?	Surgery, aimed at eradication of disease and reconstruction of the ossicular chain

BULLOUS MYRINGITIS _____

What is it?	A vesicular infection of the TM and adjacent deep canal
Causative agents?	Unknown; suspect viral because of frequent association with viral URI (in some instances *Mycoplasma pneumoniae* has been cultured)
Symptoms?	Acute, severe ear pain, low-grade fever, and bloody drainage
Otoscopic examination?	Shows large, reddish blebs on the TM and/or the wall of the meatus
Is hearing affected?	Not usually; occasional reversible sensorineural loss
Treatment?	Oral antibiotics (erythromycin if suspect *Mycoplasma*), may use topical analgesics, with resolution of symptoms usually in 36 hours

ACUTE SUPPURATIVE OTITIS MEDIA (OM)

What is it?	A bacterial infection of the middle ear, often following a viral upper respiratory infection; may be associated with a middle ear effusion
Cause?	Dysfunction of the eustachian tube that allows bacterial entry from nasopharynx; often associated with an occluded eustachian tube although it is uncertain whether this is a cause or a result of the infection
Predisposing factors?	Young age, maleness, bottle feeding, crowded living conditions (i.e., daycare), cleft palate, Down's syndrome, cystic fibrosis
Etiology?	1. *Streptococcus pneumoniae* ($\frac{1}{3}$) 2. *Hemophilus influenzae* 3. *Moraxella catarrhalis* 4. *Staphylococcus* 5. β-Hemolytic strep 6. Viral/no culture
In infants under 6 mo?	1. *Staphylococcus aureus* 2. *E. coli* 3. *Klebsiella*
Symptoms?	Otalgia, fever, decreased hearing; as many as 25% are asymptomatic
Signs?	Early, redness of the TM; later, TM bulging with loss of the normal landmarks and finally impaired TM mobility on pneumatic otoscopy
Complications?	Acute mastoiditis, meningitis, brain abscess, extradural abscess, labyrinthitis; if recurrent or chronic, OM may have adverse effects on speech and cognitive development
Treatment?	10-day course of abx; amoxicillin is first-line agent; if PCN allergic: trimethoprim-sulfamethoxazole or erythromycin
Usual course?	Symptoms usually resolve in 24–36 hours
Indications for myringotomy?	1. Persistent middle ear effusion over 3 months 2. Debilitated or immunocompromised patient 3. < 3 episodes over 6 months

SEROUS OTITIS MEDIA

What is it?	Usually an acute response to temporary ventilatory dysfunction of the eustachian tube
Precipitating factors?	Nasopharyngeal inflammation; often allergic rhinitis or the common cold
What more serious lesion may have similar presentation?	Nasopharyngeal carcinoma; be especially suspicious in the adult with prolonged unilateral serous otitis
Symptoms?	Sensation of otic fullness, tinnitus, hearing loss
Exam?	Amber-colored TM and often a visible fluid line or air bubbles behind the TM, which may be retracted with decreased mobility
Treatment?	Most cases resolve without treatment; antihistamines may help; myringotomy with aspiration of fluid has a high certainty of cure but is rarely necessary

MUCOID OTITIS MEDIA

Age group affected?	Usually seen in children
Associated with?	Chronic dysfunction of the eustachian tube, a common sequela of acute OM
**Most common cause of?	Acquired **hearing loss** in children
Symptoms?	Often asymptomatic, though impaired hearing is common
Exam?	Otoscopy may reveal a dull, retracted, immobile TM
Treatment?	Search for underlying etiology; Antihistamine-decongestant combinations are not efficacious; watch for 2–3 months for spontaneous resolution, myringotomy with tube insertion if no resolution

OTOSCLEROSIS

What is it?	A genetic disease characterized by abnormal spongy and sclerotic bone formation in the temporal bone around the footplate of the stapes, thus preventing its normal movement

Inheritance pattern?	Autosomal dominant with incomplete $\frac{1}{3}$ penetrance
Symptoms?	Painless, progressive hearing loss (may be unilateral or bilateral), tinnitus
Usual age of onset?	Second through fourth decade
Diagnosis?	Normal TM with conductive hearing loss (though may be mixed or even sensorineural if bone of cochlea is affected)
Treatment?	Frequently surgical (stapedectomy with placement of prosthesis), hearing aids, or observation; sodium fluoride may be used if a sensorineural component is present or for preoperative stabilization

FACIAL NERVE PARALYSIS

Localization of defect?	Supranuclear—paralysis of lower face only, forehead muscles spared due to bilateral corticobulbar supply Intratemporal bone—paralysis of upper and lower face, decreased tearing, altered taste, absent stapedius reflex Distal to stylomastoid foramen—paralysis of facial muscles only
Causes?	Usually from lesions of the nerve within its course through the temporal bone: Bell's palsy (see below) Trauma Cholesteatoma with erosion of facial canal Tumor (carcinoma, glomus jugulare) Zoster inflammation of geniculate ganglion (Ramsey-Hunt syndrome) Peripheral lesions are usually parotid gland tumors or facial laceration

BELL'S PALSY

What is it?	Sudden onset, unilateral facial weakness or paralysis in absence of CNS, ear, or cerebellopontine angle disease (i.e., no identifiable cause)
Clinical course?	Acute onset, with greatest muscle weakness reached within 3 weeks

Incidence?	Most common cause of unilateral facial weakness/paralysis
Pathogenesis?	Unknown; most widely accepted hypothesis is viral etiology; ischemic and immunologic factors also implicated
Common preceding event?	Upper respiratory tract infection
Signs/Sx?	Pathology is related to swelling of the facial nerve; may present with total facial paralysis, altered lacrimation, increased tearing on affected side, change in taste if region above chorda tympani is affected, dry mouth, and hyperacusis
Treatment?	Usually none is required, as most resolve spontaneously in 1 month; protect eye with drops if it cannot be closed; some advocate steroids or surgical decompression of CN VII if paralysis progresses or tests indicate deterioration
Prognosis?	Overall, 90% recover completely; if paralysis is incomplete, 95–100% will recover without sequelae

SENSORINEURAL HEARING LOSS

What is it?	Hearing loss caused by a lesion occurring in the cochlea or acoustic nerve rather than the external or middle ear
Symptoms?	Distortion of hearing, impaired speech discrimination, tinnitus
Signs?	Air conduction better than bone conduction (positive Rinne test), Weber lateralizes to the side without the defect; audiogram varies but most commonly shows greatest loss in high-frequency tones
Causes?	Aging (presbycusis)—#1 cause Acoustic injury from sudden or prolonged exposure to loud noises Congenital (maternal rubella, CMV, toxoplasmosis, syphilis) Meniere's disease

Drug/toxin-induced (abx, esp. aminoglycosides; aspirin; quinine; anticancer meds such as cisplatin; loop diuretics)

Acoustic neuroma

Pseudotumor cerebri

CNS disease (multiple sclerosis)

Endocrine disorders (diabetes, hypothyroid)

Sarcoidosis

Metabolic disorders (hyperlipoproteinemia, chronic renal failure)

Chronic otitis media

Treatment?   Hearing aids, lip reading, cochlear implant

VERTIGO

What is it?   The sensation of head movement, usually rotational

Cause?   Asymmetric neuronal activity between right and left vestibular systems

History?   Must attempt to differentiate between central and peripheral disease

Peripheral: severe vertigo, nausea, vomiting, always accompanied by horizontal or rotatory nystagmus (fast component almost always to side opposite disease), other evidence of inner ear disease (tinnitus, hearing loss); frequently associated with a previously operated ear, a chronic draining ear, barotrauma, or abdominal or head trauma

Central (brainstem or cerebellum): insidious onset, less intense and more subtle sensation of vertigo; difficulty describing the symptoms; occasionally, vertical nystagmus

Diagnostic evaluation?   Depends on probability of central vs. peripheral; need careful neurologic and otologic examinations. May need FTA/VDRL, temporal bone scans/CT/MRI, ENG, position testing, audiometric testing

Most common etiology?   Benign paroxysmal positional vertigo (BPPV); history of brief spells of severe vertigo with specific head positions

Differential diagnosis?	*Central:* vertebral basilar insufficiency (often in older patients with DJD of spine), Wallenberg syndrome, MS, epilepsy, migraine.
	Peripheral: motion sickness, syphilis, Meniere's disease, vestibular neuronitis, labyrinthitis, acoustic neuroma

MENIERE'S DISEASE

What is it?	Disorder of the membranous labyrinth causing fluctuating sensorineural hearing loss, episodic vertigo, nystagmus, tinnitus, and aural fullness
Classic triad?	Hearing loss, tinnitus, vertigo
Pathophysiology?	Obscure, but most believe excessive production/defective resorption of endolymph
Treatment?	Primarily medical: salt restriction, diuretics (thiazides), antinausea agents; occasionally diazepam is added; 80% respond to medical management
	Surgery is offered to those who fail medical treatment or who have incapacitating vertigo (60–80% effective)

VESTIBULAR NEURITIS

What is it?	Severe attack(s) of prolonged vertigo; thought to have a viral origin
Typical history?	Healthy adult (age 30–60) who has had a URI or sinusitis prior to an acute vestibular crisis characterized by severe vertigo, nausea, vomiting, and nystagmus
Course?	Symptoms usually last 3–7 days, with progressive improvement noted following a single episode; recurrences (usu. less severe) may occur in the ensuing weeks
Treatment?	IV phenothiazine given slowly will usually stop severe vertigo, nausea, and vomiting; diazepam or meclizine (vestibulosuppressives) may be helpful; mainstay of treatment is early, aggressive vestibular rehabilitation exercises once symptoms have been controlled

POSTERIOR FOSSA TUMORS

What is it?	Most commonly (90%) acoustic neuromas, which are benign schwannomas of CN VIII; less common primary tumors are meningioma, cholesteatoma, arachnoid cyst
Site most commonly affected?	Cerebellopontine angle
Early symptoms?	Tinnitus, hearing loss, vertigo
Later?	May involve CN IX, X, XI (caudal tumor growth), cerebellum by compression.
Diagnosis?	Audiometry, brainstem evoked potentials, radiology (CT and MRI)
Treatment?	Surgical resection

NOSE AND PARANASAL SINUSES

EPISTAXIS

What is it?	Bleeding from the nose
Predisposing factors?	Sinus infection, allergic or atrophic rhinitis, blood dyscrasias, tumor, environmental extremes (hot, dry climates, winters)
Usually caused by?	Rupture of superficial mucosal blood vessels (Kiesselbach's plexus if anterior bleed, sphenopalatine artery if posterior)
Most common type?	Anterior (90% of all epistaxis); usually due to trauma
Which type is more serious?	Posterior; usually in the elderly or associated with a systemic disorder (hypertension, arteriosclerosis)
Treatment?	Direct pressure; if this fails proceed to anterior nasal packing with gauze strips, followed if necessary by posterior packing with Foley catheter or lamb's wool; packs must be removed in <5 days to prevent infectious complications

ACUTE RHINITIS

What is it?	Inflammation of nasal mucous membrane
Most common cause?	Upper respiratory tract infection; rhinovirus is most common agent in adults (other nonallergic causes: nasal deformities and tumors, polyps, atrophy, immune diseases, vasomotor problems)

Symptoms?	Nasal stuffiness, rhinorrhea, sneezing, mild fever, headache, and general malaise; obstruction and thickened/purulent nasal discharge may follow.
Exam?	Swollen, erythematous nasal mucosa with a watery mucous discharge
Course/treatment?	Usually lasts 5–7 days; antihistamines and decongestants may help symptoms

ALLERGIC RHINITIS

Symptoms?	Nasal stuffiness, watery rhinorrhea, paroxysms of morning sneezing, and itching of nose, conjunctiva, or palate
Characterized by?	Early onset (before age 20), familial tendency, presence of other allergic disorders (exzema, asthma), elevated serum IgE
Exam?	Pale, boggy, bluish nasal turbinates coated with thin, clear secretions; in children, a transverse nasal crease is sometimes caused by repeated ''allergic salute''
Treatment?	Allergen avoidance, antihistamines, decongestants; steroids or sodium cromylate if severe; desensitization via allergen immunotherapy is the only ''cure''

ACUTE SINUSITIS

Typical history?	Previously healthy patient with unrelenting progression of a viral URI or allergic rhinitis beyond the normal 5–7 day course
Symptoms?	Periorbital pressure/pain, nasal obstruction, nasal/postnasal mucopurulent discharge, fatigue, fever, headache
Signs?	Tenderness over affected sinuses, pus in the nasal cavity; may also see reason for obstruction (septal deviation, spur, tight osteomeatal complex); transillumination is unreliable
Pathophysiology?	Thought to be secondary to decreased ciliary action of the sinus mucosa, and edema causing obstruction of the sinus ostia, lowering intrasinus oxygen tension and predisposing toward bacterial infection

Causative organisms?	Up to 50% have negative culture and are presumably (initially) viral; pneumococcus, *S. aureus,* group A streptococci, and *H. influenzae* are most common bacteria cultured
Treatment?	14-day course of abx (pen G, amoxicillin, Ceclor, and Augmentin commonly used), topical and systemic decongestants, and saline nasal irrigation

CHRONIC SINUSITIS

What is it?	Infection of nasal sinuses lasting longer than 4 weeks, or pattern of recurrent acute sinusitis punctuated by brief asymptomatic periods
Pathology?	Permanent mucosal changes secondary to inadequately treated acute sinusitis, consisting of mucosal fibrosis, polypoid growth, and inadequate ciliary action
Symptoms?	Chronic nasal obstruction, postnasal drip, mucopurulent rhinorrhea, low-grade facial and periorbital pressure/pain
Causative organisms?	Usually anaerobes (such as *Bacteroides, Veillonella, Rhinobacterium*); also *H. influenzae, Streptococcus* viridans
Treatment?	Try medical management with decongestant-antihistamine, topical steroids, and antibiotics; if this fails, proceed to endoscopic or external surgical intervention
What is FESS?	Functional endoscopic sinus surgery
Complications of sinusitis?	Orbital cellulitis (if ethmoid sinusitis), meningitis, epidural or brain abscess (frontal sinus), cavernous sinus thrombosis (ethmoid or sphenoid), osteomyelitis, A.K.A. Pott's puffy tumor (if frontal)

CANCER OF THE NASAL CAVITY AND PARANASAL SINUSES

Usual location?	Maxillary sinus (⅔) Nasal cavity Ethmoid sinus Rarely in frontal or sphenoid sinuses
Cell type?	Squamous cell (80%) Adenocellular (15%) Uncommon: sarcoma, melanoma

What rare tumor arises from olfactory epithelium?	Esthesioneuroblastoma; usu. arises high in the nose (cribriform plate) and is locally invasive
Signs/Sx?	Nasal obstruction, blood-tinged mucus, epistaxis most common early; localized pain, cranial nerve deficits, facial/palate asymmetry, loose teeth appear later
Diagnosis?	CT can adequately identify extent of disease and local invasion
Treatment?	Surgery ± XRT
Prognosis?	5-year survival for T1 or T2 lesions approaches 70%

JUVENILE NASOPHARYNGEAL ANGIOFIBROMA

What is it?	The most commonly encountered vascular mass found in the nasal cavity; locally aggressive but nonmetastasizing
History?	Usually adolescent males who present with nasal obstruction, recurrent severe epistaxis, possibly anosmia
Usual location?	Site of origin is roof of nasal cavity at superior margin of sphenopalatine foramen
Can transform into?	Fibrosarcoma (rare cases reported)
Diagnosis?	Carotid arteriography, CT; biopsy is contraindicated secondary to risk of uncontrollable hemorrhage
Treatment?	Surgery via lateral rhinotomy with bleeding controlled by internal maxillary artery ligation or embolization, in setting of hypotensive anesthesia; preoperative irradiation has also been used to shrink tumor

ORAL CAVITY AND PHARYNX

PHARYNGOTONSILLITIS

What is it?	Acute or chronic infection of the naso- or oropharynx and/or Waldeyer's ring of lymphoid tissue (consisting of palatine, lingual, pharyngeal tonsils and the adenoids)

Etiology?   Acute attacks can be viral (adenovirus, enterovirus, coxsackievirus; Epstein-Barr virus in infectious mononucleosis) or bacterial (group A β-hemolytic streptococci are the #1 bacterial agent); chronic tonsillitis often with mixed population, including streptococci, staphylococci, and *M. catarrhalis*

Symptoms?   *Acute*—Sore throat, fever, local lymphadenopathy, chills, headache, malaise
Chronic—Noisy mouthbreathing, speech and swallowing difficulties, apnea

Signs?   *Viral*—Injected tonsils and pharyngeal mucosa; exudate may occur, but less often than with bacterial tonsillitis
Bacterial—Swollen, inflamed tonsils with white-yellow exudate in crypts and on surface; cervical adenopathy

Diagnosis?   CBC, throat culture, monospot test

Complications?   Peritonsillar abscess (quinsy), retropharyngeal abscess (causing airway compromise), rheumatic fever, poststreptococcal glomerulonephritis (with β-hemolytic streptococci)

Treatment?   *Viral*—Symptomatic → Tylenol, warm saline gargles, anesthetic throat spray
Bacterial—10 days PCN (erythromycin if PCN-allergic)

Indications for tonsillectomy?   Sleep apnea/cor pulmonale secondary to airway obstruction, suspicion of malignancy, hypertrophy causing malocclusion, peritonsillar abscess, recurrent acute or chronic tonsillitis

Complications?   Acute or delayed hemorrhage

PERITONSILLAR ABSCESS _____

Clinical setting?   Inadequately treated recurrent acute or chronic tonsillitis

Microbiology?   Mixed aerobes and anaerobes (which may be PCN-resistant)

Site of formation?	Begins at superior pole of tonsil
Symptoms?	Severe throat pain, dysphagia, odynophagia, trismus, cervical adenopathy, fever, chills, malaise
Signs?	Bulging, erythematous, edematous tonsillar pillar; swelling of uvula and displacement to contralateral side
Treatment?	IV abx or surgical evacuation by incision and drainage; most recommend tonsillectomy after resolution of inflammatory changes

CANCER OF THE ORAL CAVITY _____

Usual cell type?	**Squamous cell** (in >90%)
Most common sites?	Tongue (30%), lip (25%), floor of mouth, gingiva, cheek, and palate
Etiology?	Linked to smoking, alcohol, and smokeless tobacco products
Frequency of	
Regional mets?	About 30%
Second primary?	About 25%
Nodal mets?	Depends on size of tumor and ranges from 10 to 60%, usually to jugular and **jugulodigastric nodes**
Distant mets?	Infrequent
Diagnosis?	Full H&P, dental assessment, may need panorex or bone scan if mandible is thought to be involved, CT/MRI for extent of tumor and nodal disease
Treatment?	Radiation and/or surgery for small lesions; localized lesions can usually be treated surgically; larger lesions require combination therapy, possible mandibulectomy and neck dissection

Prognosis?	Depends on stage and site
	    Tongue: 20–70% survival
	    Floor of mouth: 30–80% survival
	Most common cause of death in successfully treated head and neck cancer is development of a second primary (occurs in 20–40%)

SALIVARY GLAND TUMORS

Frequency of gland involvement?

Parotid gland (80%)
Submandibular gland (15%)
Minor salivary glands (5%)

Potential for malignancy?

Greatest in **minor salivary gland** tumors (80% are malignant) and least in parotid gland tumors (80% are benign); the smaller the gland, the greater the likelihood of malignancy

Differentiation of benign vs. malignant by Hx + PE?

Benign—mobile, nontender, no node involvement or facial weakness
Malignant—painful, fixed mass with evidence of local metastasis, and facial paresis/paralysis

Treatment?

Involves adequate surgical resection, sparing facial nerve if possible, neck dissection for node-positive necks
Postoperative RT if high-grade cancer, recurrent cancer, residual disease, invasion of adjacent structures, any T3 or T4 parotid tumors

Minimal diagnostic and therapeutic procedure for parotid neoplasms?

Superficial parotidectomy (resection the parotid superficial to the facial nerve)

Most common benign salivary tumor?
  Usual location?
  Clinical course?

Pleomorphic adenoma (benign mixed tumor) accounts for ⅔ of total
Parotid gland
They are well-delineated and slow growing

Second most common benign salivary gland tumor?
  Usual location?
  Describe lesion

Warthin's tumor (1% of all salivary gland tumors)
95% are found in parotid, 3% are bilateral
Slow-growing, cystic mass usually located in the tail of the superficial portion of the parotid; rarely becomes malignant

Most common malignant salivary tumor?

Mucoepidermoid carcinoma (10% of all salivary gland neoplasms)
  #1 parotid malignancy
  #2 submandibular gland malignancy

Second most common malignant salivary tumor in adults?

Adenoid cystic carcinoma
<10% of all salivary gland neoplasms
  #1 malignancy in submandibular and minor salivary glands
  #2 in parotid

LARYNX

ANATOMY _____

Define the three parts?

Glottis: begins halfway between the true and false cords (in the ventricle) and extends inferiorly 1.0 cm below the edge of the vocal folds

Supraglottis: extends from superior glottis to superior border of hyoid and tip of epiglottis

Subglottis: extends from lower border of glottis to inferior edge of cricoid cartilage

Innervation?

Via the vagus nerve: superior laryngeal and recurrent laryngeal nerves; superior laryngeal supplies sensory to supraglottis and motor to cricothyroid muscle; recurrent laryngeal supplies sensory to glottis and subglottis and motor to all remaining intrinsic laryngeal muscles

CROUP (LARYNGOTRACHEOBRONCHITIS) _____

What is it?

A viral infection of the larynx and trachea, generally affecting children (boys > girls)

Usual cause?

Parainfluenza virus***

Age group affected?

Most commonly in ages 6 mo–3 yr

Seasonal?

Yes; outbreaks most often in autumn

Precipitating events?

Usually preceded by URI

Classical symptom?

Barking (seal-like), nonproductive cough

Other symptoms?

Respiratory distress, low-grade fever

Signs?

Tachypnea, inspiratory retractions, prolonged inspiration, inspiratory stridor, expiratory rhonchi/wheezes

Differential diagnosis?

Epiglottis, bacterial tracheitis, foreign body, diphtheria, retropharyngeal abscess, peritonsillar abscess, asthma

Diagnosis?

Lateral neck x-ray shows classic ''steeple sign'' indicating subglottic narrowing; ABG may show hypoxemia + hypercapnia

Treatment?	*Keep child calm,* agitation only worsens obstruction; cool mist, steroids (controversial), aerosolized racemic EPI may be administered to reduce edema/airway obstruction
Intubation indications?	Intubate if airway obstruction is severe or if child becomes exhausted
Usual course?	Resolves in 3–4 days; secondary bacterial infection (streptococcal, staphylococcal) may require abx

EPIGLOTTITIS

What is it?	Severe, rapidly progressive infection of the epiglottis
Usual causative agent?	***Haemophilus influenzae* type B**
Age group affected?	Children 2–5 years old
Signs/Sx?	Sudden onset, high fever (40°C), "hot potato" voice, dysphagia (→ drooling), no cough, patient prefers to sit upright, **lean forward;** Patient appears toxic and stridulous
Diagnosis?	Can usually be made clinically and does *not* involve direct observation of the epiglottis (which may worsen obstruction by causing laryngospasm)
Treatment?	Involves immediate airway support via OR intubation or possibly tracheotomy; medical—steroids and IV abx against *H. influenzae* (ampicillin + chloramphenicol)

MALIGNANT LESIONS OF THE LARYNX

Incidence?	Accounts for ≈2% of all malignancies, more often in males
Most common site?	Glottis (⅔)
Second most common?	Supraglottis (⅓)
Worst prognosis?	Subglottic tumors (infrequent)
Risk factors?	Tobacco, ETOH
Pathology?	90% are squamous cell carcinoma

Symptoms?	Hoarseness, throat pain, dysphagia, odynophagia, neck mass, (referred) ear pain

Supraglottic Lesions

Usual location?	Laryngeal surface of epiglottis
Often involve?	Preepiglottic space
Extension?	Tend to remain confined to supraglottic region, though may extend to valleculae or base of tongue
Metastasis?	High propensity for nodal metastasis

Glottic Lesions

Usual location?	Anterior part of true cords
Extension?	May invade thyroid cartilage, cross midline to invade contralateral cord, or invade paraglottic space
Metastasis?	Rare nodal metastasis
Treatment?	Total or supraglottic laryngectomy, depending on location and extent of lesion; neck dissection if nodal involvement

Five-year survival for	
T1 lesions?	90%
T2 lesions?	80%
T3 lesions?	75%
T4 lesions?	30%

Neck Mass

Usual etiology in infants?	Congenital (branchial cleft cysts, thyroglossal duct cysts)
Adolescents?	Inflammatory (cervical adenitis #1), with congenital also possible
Adults?	Malignancy (squamous #1), esp. if painless and immobile
80% Rule?	In general, 80% of neck masses are **benign** in children; 80% are **malignant** in adults > 40
Seven cardinal symptoms of neck masses?	Dysphagia, odynophagia, hoarseness, stridor (signifies upper airway obstruction), globus, speech disorder, referred ear pain (via CN V, IX, or X)
Define dysphagia	Difficulty swallowing
Define odynophagia	Painful swallowing

Define Globus	Sensation of a ''lump in the throat''
Workup?	Full head + neck exam, indirect laryngoscopy, CT and MRI to search for hidden primary; **FNA for tissue Dx;** biopsy contraindicated as it has an adverse effect on survival if malignant
Differential diagnosis?	*Inflammatory:* cervical lymphadenitis, cat-scratch disease, infectious mono, infection in neck spaces *Congenital:* thyroglossal duct cyst (midline, elevates with tongue protrusion), branchial cleft cysts (lateral), dermoid cysts (midline submental), hemangioma, cystic hygroma *Neoplastic:* primary or metastatic
Treatment?	Surgical excision for congenital or neoplastic; two most important procedures for cancer treatment are radical and modified neck dissection

RADICAL NECK DISSECTION _____

What is involved?	Classically, it involves removal of: **nodes** from clavicle to mandible, **sternocleidomastoid muscle, submaxillary gland,** tail of **parotid,** internal **jugular vein, digastric muscles, stylohyoid** and **omohyoid muscles, fascia** within the anterior and posterior triangles, **CN XI,** and cervical plexus sensory nerves
Indications?	1. Presence of clinically positive nodes that likely contain metastatic cancer 2. Clinically negative neck but high probability of metastasis from a primary tumor elsewhere 3. A fixed cervical mass that is resectable
Contraindications?	1. Distant metastasis 2. Fixation to structure that cannot be removed 3. Low neck masses

MODIFIED NECK DISSECTION _____

Types?	
Type I?	Type I—spinal accessory nerve is preserved
Type II?	Type II—spinal accessory and internal jugular preserved

Type III?	Type III—spinal accessory, IJ, and sternocleidomastoid preserved
Advantages?	Increased postoperative function and decreased morbidity (esp. if bilateral), most often used in N0 lesions; these modifications are usually intraoperative decisions based on the location and extent of tumor growth
Disadvantages?	May result in increased mortality from local recurrence

FACIAL FRACTURES

MANDIBLE FRACTURES _____

Symptoms?	Gross disfigurement, pain, **malocclusion, drooling**
Signs?	Trismus, fragment mobility and lacerations of gingiva, hematoma in floor of mouth
Complications?	Malunion; nonunion; osteomyelitis; TMJ ankylosis
Treatment?	Open or closed reduction

MIDFACE FRACTURES _____

Evaluation?	Careful physical examination and CT

Classification _____

Le Fort I?	*Le Fort I:* transverse maxillary fx above the dental apices, which also traverses the pterygoid plate; palate is mobile, but nasal complex is stable

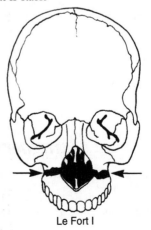

Le Fort I

Le Fort II?

Le Fort II: fx through frontal process of maxilla, through orbital floor, and pterygoid plate; midface is mobile

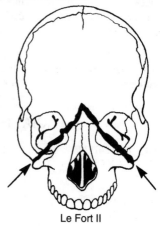

Le Fort II

Le Fort III?

Le Fort III: **complete craniofacial separation,** differs from II in that it extends through the nasofrontal suture and frontozygomatic sutures

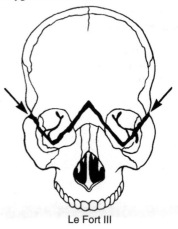

Le Fort III

ENT WARD QUESTIONS

How can you tell otitis externa from OM on PE?

Otitis externa characterized by severe pain upon manipulation of the auricle

What causes otitis media?

Majority caused by pneumococcus and *H. influenzae*

What causes otitis externa?	*Pseudomonas aeruginosa*
What do you need to consider in unilateral serous otitis?	Nasopharyngeal carcinoma
What is most common cause of facial paralysis?	**Bell's palsy,** which has an unidentified etiology
What is the single most important prognostic factor in Bell's palsy?	Whether or not the affected muscles are completely paralyzed (if not, prognosis is >95% complete recovery)
What is the classic triad of Meniere's disease?	Hearing loss, tinnitus, vertigo
What, and where, is the most common posterior fossa tumor?	Acoustic neuromas, usually occurring at the cerebellopontine angle
What is the most common site of sinus cancer?	Maxillary sinus
What tumor arises from olfactory epithelium?	Esthesioneuroblastoma
What cell type is most common in head & neck CA?	Squamous cell
What are the most important predisposing factors to head & neck cancer?	Excessive alcohol use and **tobacco** abuse of any form
Most frequent site of salivary gland tumor?	Parotid gland
Greatest proportion of salivary gland cancers?	Minor salivary glands (>75% malignant)
Classic feature of croup?	Barking, seal-like cough
Classic features of epiglottitis?	"Hot potato" voice, sitting up, **drooling,** toxic appearance, high fever, **leaning forward**
Workup of neck mass?	Do NOT biopsy; obtain tissue **via FNA,** and complete head & neck exam

41
Thoracic Surgery

DISEASES OF THE CHEST WALL

PECTUS EXCAVATUM

What is it?	Posterior curvature of the body of the sternum; "funnel chest"
Incidence?	Most common chest wall deformity
Risk factors?	Family history
Symptoms?	Usually asymptomatic, but severe deformity may lead to fatigue and increased incidence of chronic bronchitis and bronchiectasis due to impaired pulmonary expansion
Signs?	Depression, usually symmetrical, of the lower sternum with outward bowing of the costal cartilages
Diagnostic tests?	CXR will reveal severity of sternal depression and leftward displacement of the heart
Treatment?	Surgical repair of moderate-to-severe cases at age 2–4 or later if patient becomes symptomatic (exercise-induced dyspnea) or is felt to have severe disfigurement that is psychologically disabling
Prognosis?	Excellent

- Recurrence of deformity in <2% of cases
- Rarely, avascular necrosis of the sternum
- Many cases correct spontaneously before age 3

PECTUS CARINATUM

What is it?	Protrusion deformity of the anterior chest due to overgrowth of the costal cartilage; "pigeon chest"
Incidence?	10× less common than pectus excavatum

Symptoms?	Dyspnea, pulmonary infections, asthma
Signs? (2)	1. Forward buckling of the upper or lower sternum 2. Prominent use of diaphragm and accessory muscles
Treatment?	Surgical repair
Prognosis?	Excellent

THORACIC OUTLET SYNDROME

What is it?	Compression of the subclavian vessels and/or the brachial plexus at the superior outlet of the thorax

Causes? (2)	1. Various congenital anomalies, including cervical rib or abnormal fascial bands to the 1st rib
	2. Trauma:
	   a. Fracture of clavicle or 1st rib
	   b. Dislocation of humeral head
	   c. Crush injuries

Symptoms?	1. Paresthesias (neck, shoulder, arm, hand); 90% in ulnar n. distribution 2. Weakness (neural/arterial) 3. Coolness of involved extremity (arterial) 4. Edema, venous distension, discoloration (venous)
Signs?	1. Pagen–Von Schroetter syndrome—venous thrombosis leading to edema, arm discoloration, and distension of the superficial veins 2. Weak brachial and radial pulses in the involved arm 3. Hypesthesia/anesthesia 4. Occasionally, atrophy in the distribution of the ulnar nerve 5. + Adson maneuver/+ Tinsel's sign 6. Edema

What is the Adson maneuver?	Patient
	   1. Extends neck (lifts head)
	   2. Takes a deep breath
	   3. Turns head toward examined side
	Physician
	Monitors radial pulse on examined side; + test: if during maneuver the radial pulse decreases or disappears

What is Tinsel's test?	Tapping of the supraclavicular fossa produces paresthesias

Differential diagnosis?	1. Cervical spine
	    Ruptured intervertebral disk
	    Osteoarthritis
	    Spinal cord tumors
	2. Peripheral neuropathy
	3. Brachial plexus palsy
	4. Arterial
	    Aneurysm
	    Embolism
	    Occlusive disease
	    Thromboangiitis obliterans
	    Raynaud's disease
	5. Venous
	    Thrombophlebitis
	    Vasculitis, collagen disease

Treatment?	1. Physical therapy 2. Decompression of the thoracic outlet by resecting the 1st rib and cervical rib (if present) if PT fails

CHEST WALL TUMORS

Benign

Most common types?	1. Fibrous rib dysplasia 2. Chondroma 3. Osteochondroma
Treatment?	Wide excision and reconstruction with autologous or prosthetic grafts

Malignant Tumors

Most common types?	1. Fibrosarcoma 2. Chondrosarcoma 3. Osteogenic sarcoma 4. Rhabdomyosarcoma 5. Myeloma 6. Ewing's sarcoma
Treatment?	Excision as for benign tumors +/− radiation

DISEASES OF THE PLEURA

PLEURAL EFFUSION

What is it?	Fluid in the pleural space

Causes?	1. Pulmonary infections 2. Congestive heart failure 3. SLE or rheumatoid arthritis 4. Pancreatitis (sympathetic effusion) 5. Trauma 6. Pulmonary embolism 7. Renal disease 8. Cirrhosis 9. Malignancy (lymphoma/mets)
Symptoms?	Dyspnea, pleuritic chest pain
Signs?	1. Decreased breath sounds 2. Dullness to percussion 3. Egophony at the upper limit
Properties of a transudate?	1. Specific gravity <1.016 2. Protein < 3 g/dl 3. Few cells
Properties of an exudate?	1. SG > 1.016 2. Protein > 3 g/dl 3. Many cells
Key diagnostic test?	Thoracentesis (needle drainage) with studies including cytology
Treatment?	1. Pigtail catheter or thoracostomy (chest tube) 2. Treat underlying condition 3. Consider sclerosis

MESOTHELIOMA

What is it?	A primary pleural neoplasm
What are the 2 types?	1. Localized (benign or malignant) 2. Diffuse (highly malignant)
Risk factors?	1. Exposure to asbestos 2. Smoking
Symptoms?	1. Localized: pleuritic pain, joint pain and swelling, dyspnea 2. Diffuse: malaise, weight loss, cough
Signs?	Pleural effusion present in only 10–15% with local disease, almost always in diffuse disease
Diagnostic tests?	Localized: x-ray may reveal a peripheral mass, often forming an obtuse angle with the chest wall

Treatment?	Localized: surgical excision Diffuse: radiation or chemotherapy
Prognosis?	Localized: poor if tumor is malignant Diffuse: occasional long-term remissions with chemotherapy

DISEASES OF THE LUNGS

BRONCHOGENIC CARCINOMA _____

Annual incidence of lung cancer in US?	150,000 new cases
Annual deaths from lung CA?	100,000 (increasing in women); most common cancer in U.S.
#1 Risk factor?	Smoking (surprise!)
Signs/Sx?	1. Change in a chronic cough 2. Hemoptysis 3. Pleural effusion (suggests chest wall involvement) 4. Hoarseness (recurrent laryngeal nerve involvement) 5. Superior vena cava syndrome 6. Diaphragmatic paralysis (phrenic nerve involvement) 7. Usually asymptomatic until metastasis/ paraneoplastic syndrome
What is Pancoast's tumor?	Tumor at the apex of the lung or superior sulcus may involve the brachial plexus, sympathetic ganglia, and vertebral bodies, leading to pain, upper extremity weakness, and Horner's syndrome
5 most common sites of extrathoracic metastases?	1. Liver 2. Adrenals ** 3. Brain 4. Bone 5. Kidney
What are paraneoplastic syndromes?	Syndromes that are associated with tumors but which may affect distant parts of the body; they may be caused by hormones released from endocrinologically active tumors or may be of uncertain etiology

Name 5 general types of paraneoplastic syndromes	1. Metabolic: Cushing's, SIADH, hypercalcemia 2. Neuromuscular: Eaton-Lambert syndrome, cerebellar ataxia 3. Skeletal: hypertrophic osteoarthropathy 4. Dermatologic: acanthosis nigrans 5. Vascular: thrombophlebitis Trousseaus
Useful diagnostic tests?	1. Sputum cytology 2. Chest x-ray 3. Needle biopsy (if patient not an operative candidate) 4. Bronchoscopy with brushings or biopsies 5. Mediastinoscopy, mediastinotomy, scalene node biopsy, or open lung biopsy for definitive diagnosis
For each tumor listed, recall its usual site in the lung and its natural course **Squamous cell?**	⅔ occur centrally in lung hilus; may also be a Pancoast's tumor; slow growth, late metastasis; associated with smoking. **Memory hint: S**quamous = **S**entral
Adenocarcinoma?	Peripheral; rapid growth with hematogenous/nodal metastasis; associated with lung scarring
Small (oat) cell?	Central, highly malignant, usually not operable
Large cell?	Usually peripheral; very malignant
Treatment for lung CA?	Surgical resection when possible
6 contraindications to surgery?	1. **S**calene nodes positive or **S**uperior vena cava syndrome 2. **T**racheal carina involvement 3. **O**at cell carcinoma 4. **P**ulmonary function tests shows FEV1 <1 or PCO_2 >50 5. Myocardial **I**nfarction, angina, arrhythmia 6. **T**umor elsewhere (metastatic disease) Acronym: **STOP IT**
What is hypertrophic pulmonary osteoarthropathy?	Periosteal proliferation and new bone formation at the end of long bones and in bones of hand
Incidence?	Seen in 2–12% of patients with lung CA
Signs?	Associated with clubbing of fingers; Dx by x-ray of long bones revealing periosteal bone hypertrophy

CARCINOID TUMOR

What is it?	An APUD cell (amine-precursor uptake and decarboxylation) tumor of the bronchus
Natural course in lung?	Slow growing (but may be malignant)
Primary local findings?	Wheezing and atelectasis caused by bronchial obstruction/stenosis
May be confused with?	Asthma
Diagnosis?	Bronchoscopy reveals round red-yellow mass that may bleed if biopsied
Treatment?	Surgical resection (lobectomy with lymph node dissection)

SOLITARY PULMONARY NODULES (COIN LESIONS)

What are they?	Peripheral circumscribed pulmonary lesions secondary to granulomatous disease, benign neoplasms, or malignancy
What percentage are malignant?	Overall, 5–10% (but >50% malignant in smokers over 50 years old)
Is there a gender risk?	Yes; the incidence of coin lesions is 3–9 times higher in males, and malignancy is nearly twice as common
Symptoms?	Usually absent with a solitary nodule, but may include cough, weight loss, chest pain and hemoptysis
Signs?	Physical findings are uncommon; clubbing is rare; hypertrophic osteoarthropathy implies > 80% chance of malignancy
Diagnosis?	Chest x-ray
Significance of "popcorn" calcification?	Most likely benign (i.e., hamartoma)
Risk factors for malignancy?	1. Size: lesions >1 cm have a significant chance of malignancy and those >4 cm are very likely to be malignant. 2. Indistinct margins (corona radiata) 3. Documented growth on follow-up x-ray 4. Age

Lab tests?	1. TB skin tests, etc. 2. Sputum cultures are usually negative 3. Sputum cytology is diagnostic in 5–20% of cases
Other diagnostic tests?	Bronchoscopy, chest CT, mediastinoscopy, excisional biopsy
Treatment?	Surgical excision is the mainstay of treatment 1. Excisional biopsy is therapeutic for benign lesions, solitary mets, and for primary cancer in patients who are poor risks for more extensive surgery 2. Lobectomy for centrally placed lesions 3. Lobectomy with node dissection for primary cancer
Prognosis?	For malignant coin lesions <2 cm, 5-year survival is about 70%—significantly higher than for lung cancer in general
What if the patient has an SPN and pulmonary hypertrophic osteoarthropathy?	The patient has >75% chance of having a carcinoma

DISEASES OF THE MEDIASTINUM

MEDIASTINAL ANATOMY

What structures lie in the anterior mediastinum?	Thymus, ascending aorta, aortic arch, great vessels, lymph nodes
... middle mediastinum?	Heart, trachea and bifurcation, lung hila, phrenic nerves, lymph nodes
... posterior mediastinum?	Esophagus, descending aorta, thoracic duct, vagus and intercostal nerves, sympathetic trunks, azygous and hemiazygous veins, lymph nodes
Major differential for tumors of the mediastinum **Anterior mediastinum?**	The classic 4 Ts: Thyroid tumor, Thymoma, Terrible lymphoma, Teratoma; also parathyroid tumor, lipoma, vascular aneurysms
Middle mediastinum?	Lymphadenopathy (lymphoma, sarcoid, etc.), teratoma, fat pad, cysts, hernias, extension of esophageal mass, bronchogenic CA

Posterior mediastinum?	Neurogenic tumors**, lymphoma, Ao aneurysm, vertebral lesions, hernias
Differential for a neurogenic tumor?	Schwannomas (A.K.A. neurolemmoma), neurofibroma, neuroblastoma, ganglioneuroma, ganglioneuroblastoma, pheochromocytoma

PRIMARY MEDIASTINAL TUMORS

Thymoma

Where in the mediastinum?	Anterior

Teratomas

What are they?	Tumors of branchial cleft cells; the tumors contain ectoderm, endoderm, and mesoderm
Age group affected?	Usually adolescents, but can be any age
Where in the mediastinum?	Anterior
Characteristic x-ray findings?	Calcifications or teeth; tumors may be cystic
What percentage are malignant?	15%
Treatment?	Surgical excision

Neurogenic Tumors

Incidence?	Most common mediastinal tumors in all age groups
Where in the mediastinum?	Posterior, in the paravertebral gutters
What percentage are malignant?	50% in children 10% in adults
Histologic types (5)? (note cells of origin and whether benign or malignant)	1. Neurilemmoma or schwannoma (benign)—arise from Schwann cell sheaths of intercostal nerves 2. Neurofibroma (benign)—arise from intercostal nerves; These can degenerate into 3. Neurosarcoma (malignant) 4. Ganglioneuroma (benign)—from sympathetic chain 5. Neuroblastoma (highly malignant)—also from sympathetic chain

Lymphoma _____

Where in the mediastinum?	Anywhere, but most often in anterior mediastinum
What percentage of lymphomas involve mediastinal nodes?	50%
Symptoms?	Cough, fever, chest pain, weight loss, SVC syndrome, chylothorax
Diagnosis?	1. Chest x-ray, CT 2. Mediastinoscopy or mediastinotomy with node biopsy
Treatment?	Nonsurgical (chemotherapy and/or radiation)

MEDIASTINITIS _____

Acute Mediastinitis _____

What is it?	Acute suppurative mediastinal infection
Name 6 etiologies:	1. Esophageal perforation (Boerhaave's syndrome) 2. Postop wound infection 3. Head and neck infections 4. Lung or pleural infections 5. Rib or vertebral osteomyelitis 6. Distant infections
Clinical features?	Fever, chest pain, dysphagia (especially with esophageal perforation), respiratory distress, leukocytosis
Treatment?	1. Airway, Breathing, and Circulation (always 1st!) 2. Wide drainage 3. Treat primary cause 4. Antibiotics

Chronic Mediastinitis _____

What is it?	Mediastinal fibrosis secondary to chronic granulomatous infection
Most common etiology?	*Histoplasma capsulatum*
Clinical features?	50% are asymptomatic; symptoms are related to compression of adjacent structures: SVC syndrome, bronchial and esophageal strictures, constrictive pericarditis

Diagnosis?	CXR or CT may be helpful, but surgery is the best way to make the diagnosis
Treatment?	Antibiotics; surgical removal of the granulomas is rarely helpful

SUPERIOR VENA CAVA SYNDROME

What is it?	**Obstruction of the superior vena cava,** usually by extrinsic compression
#1 cause?	**Malignant tumors** cause ≈90% of the cases; lung cancer is by far the most common; other tumors include thymoma, lymphoma, and Hodgkin's disease.
Name 3 other causes	1. Chronic mediastinitis 2. Benign tumors 3. Thrombosis
Clinical manifestations?	1. Blue discoloration and puffiness of face, arms, and shoulders 2. CNS manifestations may include headache, nausea, vomiting, visual distortion, stupor, and convulsions 3. Cough, hoarseness, and dyspnea
What may aggravate symptoms?	Lying flat or bending over
What is the clinical course?	This depends on the rapidity of onset; rapid onset of severe obstruction with no time to develop collateral circulation leads to severe symptoms and possibly fatal cerebral edema; chronic onset, as in fibrosing mediastinitis, may be very insidious and mild as collateral drainage develops
Diagnosis?	1. Confirmed by measuring upper extremity venous pressure 2. Venography localizes the obstruction
Treatment?	1. Diuretics and fluid restriction 2. Prompt radiation therapy for any causative cancer 3. Surgical excision of resectable lesions 4. Surgery to bypass SVC, replace it, or recanalize the lumen 5. In chronic total obstruction, patients will gradually improve without treatment

Prognosis?	SVC obstruction itself is fatal in <5% of cases; mean survival time in patients with malignant obstruction is about 7 months

DISEASES OF THE ESOPHAGUS

ANATOMIC CONSIDERATIONS

Primary function of the UES?	Swallowing
... of the LES?	Prevention of reflux
The esophageal venous plexus drains inferiorly into the gastric veins. Why is this important?	The gastric veins are part of the portal venous system; portal hypertension can thus be referred to the esophageal veins, leading to varices

OROPHARYNGEAL DYSPHAGIA

What is it?	Improper relaxation of the upper esophageal sphincter
Describe the pathophysiology and the resulting complication	Incoordination between relaxation of the upper esophageal sphincter and contraction of the pharynx leads to eventual formation of *Zenker's diverticulum,* which is a false diverticulum (mucosa only) above the cricopharyngeus muscle
Symptoms?	Dysphagia, reflux of undigested food, left sided neck mass, halitosis
Diagnostic tests?	History and physical exam; endoscopy to rule out other esophageal disorders—must be taken with caution as not to rupture through the diverticulum
Treatment?	1. Myotomy of cricopharyngeus muscle 2. Excision of diverticulum
What muscle is involved with a Zenker's diverticulum?	**Cricopharyngeus muscle**

ACHALASIA

What is it?	Absence of peristalsis in the body of the esophagus, combined with the failure of the lower esophageal sphincter to relax during swallowing
Proposed etiologies?	1. Ganglionic dysfunction 2. Chagas' disease in South America

Associated long-term condition?	Esophageal carcinoma secondary to Barrett's esophagus due to food stasis
Symptoms?	Dysphagia for both solids and liquids, followed by regurgitation; dysphagia for liquids is worse.
Diagnostic tests?	1. Radiographic contrast studies reveal dilated esophageal body with narrowing inferiorly 2. Motility studies reveal increased pressure in the LES and failure of the LES to relax during swallowing
Treatment?	1. Balloon dilation of LES 2. Myotomy of the lower esophagus and LES 3. Medical treatment of reflux

DIFFUSE ESOPHAGEAL SPASM

A.K.A.?	"Nutcracker esophagus"
What is it?	Strong, nonperistaltic contractions of the esophageal body; sphincter function is normal
Associated condition?	Gastroesophageal reflux
Symptoms?	Spontaneous chest pain that radiates to the back, ears, neck, jaw, or arms
Differential diagnosis?	1. Angina pectoris 2. Psychoneurosis
Diagnostic tests?	1. Motility studies reveal repetitive, high-amplitude contractions with normal sphincter response 2. Upper GI may be normal, but 50% show segmented spasms or corkscrew esophagus
Treatment?	1. Medical treatment (antireflux measures, Ca blockers, nitrates) 2. Long esophagomyotomy in refractory cases

ESOPHAGEAL REFLUX

What is it?	Reflux of gastric contents into the lower esophagus due to the decreased function of the LES

Name 4 associations

1. Sliding hiatal hernia
2. Tobacco and alcohol
3. Scleroderma
4. Decreased endogenous gastrin production

Symptoms?

Substernal pain, heartburn, regurgitation; *symptoms are worse when patient is supine and after meals*

Diagnosis?

1. pH probe in the lower esophagus reveals acid reflux
2. EGD shows esophagitis
3. Manometry reveals decreased LES pressure
4. Barium swallow

Treatment?

1. Usually medical: H2-blockers; antacids; metoclopramide, which raises LES pressure and speeds gastric emptying
2. Elevate head of bed

4 complications that require surgery?

1. Failure of medical therapy
2. Esophageal strictures
3. Progressive pulmonary insufficiency secondary to documented nocturnal aspiration
4. Barrett's esophagus

What is the surgical procedure?

Wrapping the gastric fundus around the lower esophagus to increase the sphincter tone (the most common procedure is the Nissen fundoplication)

What is Barrett's esophagus?

Replacement of lower esophageal squamous epithelium with columnar epithelium secondary to reflux

Significance?
Treatment?

This is a premalignant lesion
People with significant reflux should be followed with regular EGDs with biopsies, H2-blockers, and antireflux precautions; most believe that patients with severe dysplasia should undergo esophagectomy

ESOPHAGEAL STRICTURES

Caustic Strictures

Agents that may cause strictures if ingested?

Lye, oven cleaners, drain cleaners

Diagnosis?

Usually by history; EGD is clearly indicated early on to assess the extent of damage; scope to level of severe injury only

Treatment?	1. Neutralizing agents
	2. **Do *not* induce emesis**
	3. Corticosteroids (controversial), antibiotics (cover mouth flora)
	4. Upper GI at 10–14 days
	5. If a stricture has developed, then dilation is indicated
	6. In severe cases, esophagectomy with colon interposition or gastric pull-up

Reflux Strictures

Describe a 2-step surgical approach to treatment	1. Dilation of the stricture
	2a. If dilation is successful, then fundoplication procedure
	2b. If dilation is unsuccessful, then resection and reconstruction using stomach or bowel
Why does the esophagus heal so poorly from primary anastomosis?	There is no serosa and limited blood supply

ESOPHAGEAL CARCINOMA

What are the 2 main types?	1. Squamous cell CA in most of the esophagus
	2. AdenoCA at the GE junction
Age and gender distribution?	Most common in the 6th decade of life; men predominate
Etiologic factors (4)?	1. Tobacco
	2. Alcohol
	3. GE reflux
	4. Barrett's esophagus
Symptoms?	Dysphagia, weight loss
Diagnosis?	1. Upper GI localizes tumor
	2. EGD obtains biopsy and assesses resectability
	3. Full metastatic work-up (CXR, bone scan, CT)
Treatment?	Total thoracic esophagectomy with gastric pull-up or colon interposition
Prognosis?	Poor: surgery affords <15% survival at 5 years; if there are no demonstrable metastases, survival may reach 30%

CARDIOVASCULAR/THORACIC WARD QUESTIONS

Five ways you can increase cardiac output?

1. Iontropes
2. Chronotropic
3. Increase preload
4. Decrease afterload
5. Improve heart compliance

Side effect of protamine?

Hypotension

What is an Austin Flint murmur?

Disputed, either vibration of mitral valve secondary to regurgitant flow or filtered murmur of AI heard at apex

Where is the least oxygenated blood in the body?

Coronary sinus

Name four tumors of the anterior medistinum?

Four Ts
1. Thymomas
2. Teratomas
3. Thyroid tumor
4. Terrible lymphomas

Your patient with AS no longer has a murmur, are you worried?

Yes, not enough flow to generate a murmur

Point to the left middle lobe on this radiograph

There is no left middle lobe, the lingula is the equivalent of the right middle lobe

Indications for CABG?

1. Left main coronary dz
2. Triple vessel disease
3. Unstable/disabling angina not responsive to medical Rx
4. Postinfarct angina
5. Damage to coronary during cardiac cath
6. Disabling/refractory angina

Classic locations for aspiration pneumonia?

RUL—posterior segment
RLL—superior segments

What electrolyte must one watch during diuresis after cardiopulmonary bypass?

K^+

How does one follow extent/ progress of postbypass diuresis?

Daily weight!

During a CABG, what can one use in place of the saphenous Vein?

Internal mammary (IMA), inferior epigastric vessels, gastroepiploic vessels; *Note:* prosthetic material cannot be used!

What is a sleeve resection?   Resection of a ring segment of bronchus (with tumor inside) and then end-to-end anastomosis of the remaining ends, allowing salvage of lower lobe

What is Tietze's syndrome?   Nonsuppurative inflammation of the costochondral cartilage—painful and of unknown etiology

What is the most common cause of a cardiac tumor?   Mets!

EKG signs of
  Atrial fibrillation?   Irregularly irregular
  Ventricular aneurysm?   ST elevation
  Ischemia?   ST elevation/ST depression/Q waves/flipped t-waves

  Pericarditis?   ST elevation throughout leads
  Wolff-Parkinson-White   Delta wave = slurred upswing on QRS
  1st degree A-V block?   Prolonged P-R interval > 0.2 sec
  2nd degree A-V block?   Dropped QRS; not all p waves transmit to produce ventricular contraction

  Wenckebach phenomenon?   2nd degree block with progressive delay in P-R interval prior to dropped beat

  3rd degree A-V block?   Complete A-V disassociation; p wave and QRS random

What is Mondor's disease?   Thrombophlebitis of the thoracoepigastric veins

What is a VAD?   Ventricular Assist Device

How does a IABP work?   The intraaortic balloon pump has a balloon tip resting in the aorta; the balloon inflates in diastole increasing diastolic blood pressure and coronary blood flow; in systole the balloon deflates, creating a negative pressure lowering afterload and increasing systolic blood pressure

42
Cardiovascular Surgery

Stroke volume (SV)	ml of blood pumped/heart beat
Cardiac output (CO)	Heart rate × stroke volume
Ejection fraction	SV/end diastolic volume (nl 55–70%)
Compliance	Change in volume/change in pressure
SVR	Systemic vascular resistance

$$\frac{BP - CVP}{CO} \times 80$$

Preload	Left ventricle end diastolic pressure or volume
Afterload	Arterial resistance the heart pumps against
PVR	Pulmonary vascular resistance

$$\frac{PA - LA}{CO} \times 80$$

ACQUIRED HEART DISEASE

CORONARY ARTERY DISEASE (CAD)

What is it?	Atherosclerotic occlusive lesions of the coronary arteries (aa); segmental nature makes coronary artery bypass grafting possible
Incidence?	Number one killer in the western world; >50% is triple vessel disease involving the LAD, circumflex, and right coronary aa
Symptoms?	If ischemia occurs (low flow, vasospasm, thrombus formation, plaque rupture or a combination), patient may experience: chest pain; crushing, substernal shortness of breath; nausea/upper abdominal pain; sudden death; or may be asymptomatic
Who classically gets "silent" MIs?	Diabetics (autonomic dysfunction)

Risk factors?	1. HTN 2. Smoking 3. High (>240) cholesterol/lipids 4. Obesity 5. Diabetes mellitus 6. Family hx

Dx tests?	1. Exercise stress testing (± thallium)
	2. Echocardiography
	  • localize dyskinetic wall segments
	  • valvular dysfunction
	  • estimate ejection fraction
	3. Cardiac catheterization with coronary angiography and left ventriculography (definitive test)

Rx?	Medical therapy (beta blockers, calcium channel blockers), angioplasty (PTCA), surgical therapy: CABG
Prognosis?	About 90% survival at 5 years

CABG

What is it?	*C*oronary *A*rtery *B*ypass *G*raft
Indications?	1. Left main disease 2. Three-vessel disease (main arteries—not branches) 3. Unstable angina or disabling angina unresponsive to medical therapy 4. Postinfarct angina 5. Coronary artery rupture, dissection, thrombosis p PTCA
Procedure?	1–10 aa grafted (usually 3–6); internal mammary pedicle graft and saphenous vein free graft most often used; (IMA 95% 10-year patency vs. 70% with saphenous) procedure done under CPB
Other vessels occasionally used for grafting?	Gastroepiploic and inferior epigastric veins
Complications?	1. MI 2. Infection 3. Hemorrhage
Operative mortality?	1–2% for elective CABG (vs. 25% for acute MI)

CARDIOPULMONARY BYPASS (CPB)

What is it?

Pump and oxygenation apparatus remove blood from SVC and IVC and return it to aorta, bypassing heart & lungs, allowing cardiac arrest for open heart procedures, heart transplant, lung transplant or heart-lung transplant as well as procedures on the proximal great vessels

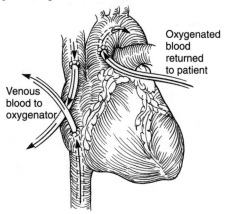

Oxygenated blood returned to patient

Venous blood to oxygenator

Procedure?

Roller pump provides nonpulsatile flow (pulse pressure <20 mm Hg); this causes no apparent problems

Anticoagulation?

Yes, just before and during procedure, with heparin

How is anticoagulation reversed?

Protamine

5 ways to manipulate cardiac output after bypass?

1. Preload—fluids
2. Inotropic state—dobutamine/epi and VAD as last resort
3. Afterload—vasodilators, heat, IABP
4. Rate, rhythm—pacer, antiarrhythmics
5. Compliance = rule out tamponade

Complications?

1. Trauma to formed blood elements (especially thrombocytopenia and platelet dysfunction)
2. Pancreatitis (low flow)
3. Heparin rebound
4. CVA
5. Failure to wean from bypass
6. Technical complications (operative technique)
7. MI

What is heparin rebound?	Increased anticoagulation after bypass due to increased heparin levels, as increase in peripheral blood flow after bypass returns heparin residual that was in the peripheral tissues
Method of lowering SVR after bypass?	Warm the patient

AORTIC STENOSIS (AS)

What is it?	Destruction and calcification of valve leaflets resulting in obstruction of LV outflow
Causes?	1. Calcification of bicuspid Ao valve 2. Rheumatic fever 3. Acquired calcific aortic stenosis (7th–8th decades)
Symptoms?	1. Angina (*3 years) 2. Syncope (*2 years) 3. CHF (*1 year) 4. Often asymptomatic until late (*life expectancy if untreated) Mnemonic: **A**ortic **S**tenosis **C**omplications (**A**ngina **S**yncope **C**HF)—3,2,1
Signs?	1. Murmur: crescendo-decrescendo systolic 2nd right ICS with radiation to the carotids 2. LV heave or lift due to LV hypertrophy
Lab tests?	1. Echocardiography 2. Cardiac cath—needed to plan operation
Rx?	Valve replacement with tissue or mechanical prosthesis if patient is symptomatic or valve cross-sectional area <1.0 cm^2 (normal 2.5–3.5 cm^2)
Pros/cons of mechanical valve?	Mechanical valve is more durable, but requires lifetime anticoagulation

AORTIC INSUFFICIENCY (AI)

What is it?	Incompetency of Ao valve
Causes?	1. Bacterial endocarditis (*Staphylococcus aureus, Streptococcus* viridans) 2. Rheumatic fever 3. Annular ectasia due to collagen vascular disease (especially Marfan's)

Predisposing conditions?	Bicuspid aortic valve
Symptoms?	1. Palpitations due to arrhythmias and dilated LV
	2. Dyspnea/orthopnea due to LV failure
	3. Angina due to decreased diastolic BP and coronary flow (*Note:* most coronary blood flow occurs during diastole and aorta rebound)
Signs?	1. Murmur: blowing, decrescendo diastolic @ LSB
	2. Austin-Flint murmur: reverberation of regurgitant flow on mitral valve
	3. Increased pulse pressure: "pistol shots," "water-hammer" pulse palpated over peripheral aa
Dx tests?	1. CXR: increasing heart size can be used to follow progression
	2. Echo
	3. Cath (definitive)
Rx?	Aortic valve replacement indicated with onset of CHF; digitalis may help the clinical picture but should not delay surgery as LV dilation is progressive; permanent injury to the LV can occur if AI left unRXD
Prognosis?	Low operative risk; surgery gives symptomatic improvement and improves longevity

MITRAL STENOSIS (MS)

What is it?	Calcific degeneration and narrowing of mitral valve due to rheumatic fever in most cases
Symptoms?	1. Dyspnea due to increased LA pressure causing pulmonary edema (i.e., CHF)
	2. Hemoptysis (rarely life-threatening)
	3. Hoarseness due to dilated LA impinging on the recurrent laryngeal nerve
Signs?	1. Murmur: crescendo diastolic rumble at apex
	2. Irregular pulse from A-fib due to dilated LA
	3. Stroke due to systemic emboli from LA (A-fib and obstructed valve allows blood to pool in the LA and can lead to thrombus formation)

Dx tests?	1. Echo 2. Cath
Rx?	1. Open commissurotomy: open heart operation with CPB where valve is cut 2. Balloon valvuloplasty: percutaneous, if unsuccessful requires operation 3. Valve replacement
Prognosis?	>80% well at 10 years with successful operation

MITRAL REGURGITATION (MR)

What is it?	Incompetence of mitral valve due to
Causes?	1. Severe mitral valve prolapse (some prolapse present in 5% of the population with female > male) 2. Rheumatic fever 3. Post-MI due to papillary mm dysfunction/rupture 4. Ruptured chordae
Most common cause?	**Ruptured chordae**/papillary muscle dysfunction
Symptoms?	Often insidious and late: dyspnea, palpitations, fatigue
Signs?	Murmur: holosystolic, apical radiating to axilla
Indications for Rx?	Indications for surgery differ from those for MS; in MR, depend more on cath and echo than symptoms (increasing regurgitation, decreasing EF, etc.) *Note:* EF first increases in MR; therefore, normal EF may actually indicate decompensation
Rx?	1. Valve replacement 2. Annuloplasty: suture a prosthetic ring to the dilated valve annulus
What is a normal ejection fraction?	55–70%

ARTIFICIAL VALVE PLACEMENT

What is it?	Replacement of damaged valves with tissue or mechanical prosthesis

Types of valves?	1. Tissue: glutaraldehyde-fixed porcine valves deteriorate over time (about 20% require replacement in 10 years), however do not require long-term anticoagulation; contraindicated in children, due to calcification
	2. Mechanical: can last for the life of the patient, but require lifelong anticoagulation; contraindicated in those with bleeding tendency (PUD, ETOH abuse, pregnancy (coumadin = teratogenic, etc.)
Operative mortality?	1–5% in most series
Postop complications?	1. Valve failure
	2. Valve deterioration: especially rapid calcification of tissue valves in children
	3. Hemorrhagic complications in anticoagulated patients (1% per year)
	4. Thromboembolic—2–5% per patient-year, even with adequate anticoagulation
	5. Conduction abnormalities due to proximity of valvular suture lines to conduction system (especially mitral valve and bundle of His)

INFECTIOUS ENDOCARDITIS

What is it?	Microbial infection of heart valves
Predisposing conditions?	Preexisting valvular lesion, procedures that lead to bacteremia/IV drug use
Common causative agents?	—*Streptococcus* viridans: assoc with abnormal valves —*Staphylococcus aureus:* assoc with IV drug use —*Staphylococcus epidermis:* assoc with prosthetic valves
Symptoms/Signs?	Referable to specific valve involved Physical exam:
	1. Murmur, new or changing
	2. Petechiae
	3. Splinter hemorrhage—fingernails
	4. Roth spots—on retina
	5. Osler nodes—raised, *painful* on soles & palms (*O*sler = *O*uch!)
	6. Janeway lesions—similar but flat and *painless* (Jane*way* = pain *away*)

Dx tests?	1. Echo
	2. Serial blood cultures (definitive)
Rx?	Prolonged IV therapy with bactericidal abx to which infecting organisms are sensitive
Prognosis?	Infection can progress to require valve replacement

CONGENITAL HEART DISEASE

VENTRICULAR SEPTAL DEFECT (VSD) _____

Claim to infamy?	Most common congenital heart defect
What is it?	Failure of ventricular septum to completely close; *80% involve the membranous portion of the septum;* this results in L to R shunt, increased pulmonary blood flow, and CHF if pulm:systemic flow > 2:1
What is Eisenmenger's syndrome?	Pulmonary HTN that develops due to chronic changes in pulmonary arterioles and increased R heart pressures; cyanosis develops when the shunt reverses (becomes R to L across the VSD)
Rx for ES?	Only option is heart-lung transplant, otherwise untreatable
Incidence of VSD?	30% of heart defects (most common defect)

PATENT DUCTUS ARTERIOSUS (PDA) _____

What is it?	Physiologic R to L shunt in fetal circulation connecting PA to aorta bypassing fetal lungs; often this shunt persists in the neonate
Factors preventing closure?	1. Hypoxia
	2. Increased prostaglandins
Symptoms?	Often asymptomatic
	1. Poor feeding
	2. Respiratory distress
	3. CHF with respiratory infections
Signs?	Acyanotic unless other cardiac lesions are present; murmur: *continuous* "machinery" murmur
Dx test?	1. Physical exam
	2. Echo (to r/o associated defects)
	3. Cath—seldom required

Rx

   Medical?   Indomethacin is a NSAID: prostaglandin
(PG) inhibitor (PG keeps PDA open)

   Surgical?   Ligation electively at 1–2 years, but if CHF
occurs, operate acutely

Prognosis?   Surgically curable lesion

TETRALOGY OF FALLOT (TOF)

What is it?   Malalignment of infundibular septum in early
development leading to characteristic tetrad:

                                    1. Pulmonary stenosis/obstruction of RV
outflow
                                    2. Overriding aorta
                                    3. RV hypertrophy
                                    4. VSD

Symptoms?   Hypoxic spells (squatting behavior increases
SVR and increases pulmonary blood flow)

Signs?   1. Cyanosis
                                    2. Clubbing
                                  3. Murmur: SEM at left 3rd ICS

Dx tests?   1. CXR: small "boot-shaped" heart and
decreased pulmonary blood flow
                                  2. Cardiac cath (definitive)

Prognosis?   90% success rate for surgical correction

What is IHSS?   Idiopathic hypertrophic subaortic stenosis

Presentation?   Can present with sudden death due to

                                    1. Arrhythmias
                                  2. Syncope
                                  3. CHF

COARCTATION OF THE AORTA

What is it?   Narrowing of thoracic aorta ± intraluminal
"shelf" (infolding of the media); usually
found near ductus/ligamentum arteriosum

Note 3 types   1. Preductal
                                        —fatal in infancy if untreated
                                  2. Juxtaductal
                                    3. Postductal

What percentage are assoc with other cardiac defects?	60%—bicuspid aortic valve most common
What is the major route of collateral circulation?	Subclavian a. to IMA to the intercostals to the descending aorta
Incidence?	10–15% of defects
Symptoms?	1. Headache 2. Epistaxis 3. LE fatigue → claudication

Signs?	• Pulses: decreased lower extremity pulses
	• Murmurs:
	    1. *Systolic*—due to turbulence across coarctation, often radiating to infrascapular region
	    2. *Continuous*—due to dilated collaterals
	• Other signs that can be assoc with fatal consequences:
	    1. CHF
	    2. Ao dissection
	    3. Intracranial aneurysmal rupture (due to HTN)
	    4. Bacterial endocarditis

Dx tests?	1. CXR
	    a. "3" sign is Ao knob, coarct, and dilated poststenotic aorta
	    b. Rib notching is bony erosion due to dilated intercostal collaterals
	2. Cath with aortography
	3. Ultrasound with Doppler

Rx?	Surgery 1. Resection with end-to-end anastomosis 2. Patch graft 3. Subclavian a. flap (favored in infants)
Surgical indications?	1. Symptomatic patient 2. Asymptomatic patient > 3–4 years
Postop complications?	1. Paraplegia 2. "Paradoxical" HTN (postop) 3. Mesenteric necrotizing panarteritis (GI bleeding)
Prognosis?	Untreated life expectancy: 30–40 years
Long-term concerns?	Ao dissection, HTN

TRANSPOSITION OF THE GREAT VESSELS _____

What is it?	Aorta originates from RV and PA from LV; incompatible with life unless patent PDA, ASD, or VSD to allow communication between the L and R circulations
Incidence?	5–8% of defects
Signs/Symptoms?	Most common lesion that presents with cyanosis and CHF in neonatal period (>90% by day 1)
Dx tests?	1. CXR: "egg-shaped" heart contour 2. Cath (definitive)
Rx?	Arterial switch operation

EBSTEIN'S ANOMALY _____

What is it?	Tricuspid valve is placed abnormally low in RA, forming a large RA and a small RV; this leads to tricuspid regurgitation and decreased RV output
Risk factors?	400× increased risk if mother has taken lithium

VASCULAR RINGS _____

What are they?	Many types; represent an anomalous development of Ao/Pa from embryonic aortic arch that surround and obstruct trachea/esophagus
Signs/symptoms?	Most prominent is stridor due to tracheal compression

CYANOTIC HEART DISEASE _____

Causes?	5 "T's" of cyanotic heart disease: Tetralogy of Fallot Truncus arteriosus TAPVR (totally anomalous pulm venous return) Tricuspid atresia Transposition of the great vessels

ADDITIONAL CARDIAC-RELATED TOPICS

POSTPERICARDIOTOMY SYNDROME

What is it?	Pericarditis after pericardiotomy (unknown etiology), occurs weeks to 3 months postop
Symptoms/signs?	1. Fever 2. Chest pain 3. Malaise 4. Pericardial friction rub
Rx?	NSAIDs, rarely steroids
What is pericarditis after a MI called?	Dressler's syndrome

CARDIAC TUMORS

Most common benign lesion?	**Myxoma** in adults, commonly found in LA with pedunculated morphology (60–80% of primary cardiac tumors)
Most common malignant tumor in children?	Rhabdomyosarcoma

DISEASES OF THE GREAT VESSELS

What is anterior spinal artery syndrome?	Syndrome characterized by a. Paraplegia b. Incontinence (bowel/bladder) c. Pain and temp sensation loss
Cause?	Occlusion of the great radicular a. of **Adamkiewicz,** which is one of the intercostal/lumbar aa from T8 to L4; seen after resection of Ao aneurysms

AORTIC DISSECTION

What is it?	Separation of the walls of the aorta due to an intimal tear and disease of the tunica media; a false lumen is formed and a "reentry" tear may occur, resulting in "double-barrel" aorta
What are the types of aortic dissection?	DeBakey classification: I. Involves ascending and descending Ao II. Ascending Ao III. Descending Ao

Stanford classification:

Type A: ascending Ao—needs operation
Type B: descending Ao—nonoperative
    except for complications

Etiology?

1. HTN—most important
2. Marfan's syndrome
3. Bicuspid Ao valve
4. Coarctation of Ao
5. Cystic medial necrosis

Signs/symptoms?

Abrupt onset of severe chest pain, often
radiating/tearing to the back; onset typically
more abrupt than in MI; the pain can migrate
as the dissection progresses; patient describes
a "tearing pain"

Note 3 other sequelae

1. Cardiac tamponade; Beck's triad—distant
   heart sounds, increased CVP with JVD,
   decreased blood pressure
2. Aortic insufficiency—diastolic murmur
3. Aortic arterial branch occlusion/shearing
   leading to ischemia in the involved
   circulation (i.e., unequal pulses, CVA,
   paraplegia, renal insufficiency, bowel
   ischemia, claudication)

Dx tests?

1. CXR
       a. widened mediastinum
       b. pleural effusion
2. Echo
3. CT
4. Aortography (definitive gold standard!)

**What is a dissecting aortic
aneurysm?**

A misnomer! not an aneurysm!

Rx?

Types I & II (A.K.A. type A)—surgical
because of

1. Ao insufficiency
2. Compromise of cerebral and coronary
   circulation
3. Tamponade
4. Rupture

Type III—medical unless complicated by
rupture or significant occlusions. (A.K.A.
type B)

Preop?	Control BP with sodium nitroprusside and β-blockers
Postop?	Lifetime control of BP and following of Ao size
What is the Edwards procedure?	Replace the ascending Ao with a graft and replace the Ao valve; with reimplantation of coronaries
Possible cause of MI in patient with aortic dissection?	Dissection involves coronary arteries

43
Transplant Surgery

DEFINITIONS

Autograft?

Same individual is donor and recipient

Isograft?

Donor and recipient are genetically identical (identical twins)

Allograft?

Donor and recipient genetically dissimilar but of the same species

Xenograft?

Donor and recipient belong to different species

Orthotopic?

Donor organ placed in anatomic position (liver, heart)

Heterotopic?

Donor organ placed in different anatomic position (kidney, pancreas)

Paratopic?

Donor organ is placed close to original organ

BASIC IMMUNOLOGY

What are histocompatibility antigens?

Distinct (genetically inherited) cell surface proteins encoded on chromosome 6 at HLA locus

Why are they important?

They are targets (class I antigens) and initiators (class II antigens) of immune response to donor tissue—i.e., key in distinguishing self from nonself

Which cells have
   Class I antigens?

All cells

   Class II antigens?

Primarily macrophages, but also B cells and some activated T cells

What is the MHC called in humans?

HLA—human leucocyte antigen

   Location?

Short arm of chromosome 6

   Codes for?

Class I, II, and III antigens

C*ELLS*

T Cells

Source?	Thymus
Function?	Cell-mediated immunity—reject; w/o T cells, no rejection
Types?	Th (CD4): *h*elper T, help B cells become plasma cells Ts (CD8): *s*uppressor T, regulate immune response Tc (CD8): *c*ytotoxic T, kill cell by direct contact

B Cells

Precursors of?	Plasma (antibody-producing) cells
Function?	Humoral immunity

Macrophage

Definition?	A monocyte in parenchymal tissue
Function?	Process foreign protein and present it to other lymphoid cells, also ''eats stuff''

IMMUNOSUPPRESSION

Who needs to be immunosuppressed?	All recipients (except auto- or isograft)

What drugs are used for immunosuppression?
    3 major ones?
    2 others?
    new one?
	
	Corticosteroids, azathioprine, cyclosporine
	MALG, OKT3, ATG
	FK-506

What is the advantage to ''triple therapy''?	Use three immunosuppressive drugs and thereby can use lower doses of each and decrease the toxic side effects of each

C*ORTICOSTEROIDS*

Most commonly used in transplants?	Prednisone
Function?	Primarily blocks production of IL-1 by macrophage and stabilizes lysosomal membrane of macrophage
Toxicity?	''Cushingoid,'' alopecia, striae, HTN, diabetes, pancreatitis, ulcer dz, osteomalacia, aseptic necrosis (especially of the femoral head)

Relative potency of
Cortisol?	1
Prednisone?	4
Methylprednisolone?	5
Dexamethasone?	25

AZATHIOPRINE—AZA (IMURAN)

Function?	Prodrug that is cleaved into mercaptopurine; inhibits synthesis of DNA & RNA, so decreased cellular production
Toxicity?	Toxic to bone marrow (leukopenia + thrombocytopenia), hepatotoxic, pancreatitis
When lower dose of AZA?	When WBC <4
Drug interaction?	Decrease dose if patient also on allopurinol, since allopurinol inhibits the enzyme xanthine oxidase which is necessary for the breakdown of azathioprine

CYCLOSPORINE—CSA

Function?	Inhibits the production of IL-2 by Th cells and monocytes

Toxicity?	1. Nephrotoxic (dose-dependent, reversible)
	2. Elevated LFTs in 50%
	3. Neurotoxic
	    tremor 50%
	    seizures 5%
	4. HTN
	5. Gum hypertrophy
	6. Hirsutism
	7. Hyperkalemia

What drugs ↑ CSA levels?	Diltiazem Ketoconazole Erythromycin
What is the drug of choice for HTN due to CSA?	Clonidine

MALG/ATG (MINNESOTA ANTILYMPHOBLAST/ANTITHYMOCYTE GLOBULIN)

Function?	An antibody against lymphoblasts and thymocytes
How made?	Inject human lymphoblasts and lymphocytes into a horse or rabbit and retrieve antibodies
Toxicity?	Thrombocytopenia, leukopenia, serum sickness, rigors, fever, anaphylaxis, increased risk of viral infection

OKT3 _____

Function?	Antibody that binds to CD3 receptor (a specific antigen on T cells)
Problem?	Because it is monoclonal, blocking antibodies develop; so less effective each time it is used

What drug acts at the following sites?

What drug acts at:

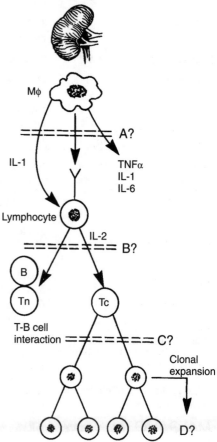

A. **Site of action of?**   A. Corticosteroids

B. **Site of action of?**   B. Cyclosporine

C. **Site of action of?**   C. Azathioprine

D. **Site of action of?**   D. MALG/ATG

MATCHING OF DONOR AND RECIPIENT

ABO cross-match?	Same as in blood typing
Universal donor?	O
Universal recipient?	AB
When do you cross bloodlines?	Only in an EMERGENCY liver transplant!
Lymphocytotoxic cross-match	
Purpose?	Test for HLA Abs in serum; most important in kidney, heart, pancreas transplants
How?	Mix recipient serum with donor lymphocyte and rabbit complement
HLA match?	Done for all organs; 6 antigen matches must be offered to potential recipient

REJECTION

How many methods of rejection?	Basically 2—humoral and cell-mediated
Name the types of rejection	Hyperacute, acute, chronic
Time courses by type?	Hyperacute—immediate in OR Acute—weeks to months post tx Chronic—months to years
What happens in hyperacute?	Antigraft Abs in recipient recognize foreign Ag immediately after blood perfuses organ
Rx for hyperacute?	Remove transplanted organ, *pronto*
Rx for acute rejection?	High-dose steroids
Rx for chronic rejection?	Not much
Note mechanism of rejection:	
Hyperacute?	Secondary to recipient preformed antibodies to donor ABO or HLA Ag
Acute?	Humoral and cellular immunity
Chronic?	Humoral and cellular immunity
Clinical signs of acute rejection?	Fever, graft tenderness, decreased function of graft = increase bilirubin in oltx and increase in serum creatinine in renal tx, edema

ORGAN PRESERVATION

Storage temp of organ?	4°C—keep on ice in Playmate cooler
Why keep it cold?	Cold decreases the rate of chemical reactions; decreased energy use minimizes effects of hypoxia and ischemia

What is U-W solution?	University of Wisconsin solution; used to perfuse organ prior to removal from donor
What is in it?	Potassium phosphate, buffers, starch, steroids, insulin, electrolytes, adenosine
Why use it?	Lengthens organ preservation time

MAXIMUM TIME BETWEEN HARVEST AND TRANSPLANT OF ORGAN ____

Heart?	4–6 hr
Lung?	6–8 hr
Pancreas?	24 hr
Liver?	24 hr
Kidney?	Up to 48 hr

KIDNEY TRANSPLANT

HISTORY _____

Year of 1st transplant in man?	1954
By whom?	Dr. J.E. Murray—1990 Nobel Prize in Medicine
Indications for xplant?	Irreversible renal failure due to

1. Glomerulonephritis (#1 cause)
2. Pyelonephritis
3. Polycystic kidney disease
4. Malignant HTN
5. Reflux pyelonephritis
6. Goodpasture's syndrome (anti–basement membrane)
7. Congenital renal hyperplasia
8. Fabry's disease
9. Alport's syndrome
10. Renal cortical necrosis
11. Damage due to IDDM

Define renal failure	GFR < 20–25% of normal; as GFR drops to ≤5–10% of normal, uremic symptoms begin (lethargy, seizures, neuropathy, electrolyte disorders)

STATISTICS _____

Sources of donor kidneys?	70% Cadaveric 30% Living related donor (LRD)
Survival for **Cadaveric?**	85% at 1 yr if HLA matched 80% at 1 yr if not HLA matched 75% graft survival at 3 yr

LRD?	90–95% patient survival at 3 yr 75–85% graft survival at 3 yr
Tests for compatibility?	ABO, HLA typing
If have of choice of donor kidney—L or R?	Choose L—longer renal vein = easier anastomosis
Placement of kidney, hetero- or orthotopic? **Why?**	Heterotopic—retroperitoneal in RLQ or LLQ above inguinal ligament Preserve native kidneys, easy access to iliac vessels, ureter close to bladder, easy to bx
Placement of ureter?	Put submucosally through bladder wall—decrease reflux
Why keep native kidneys?	Increased morbidity to take out
Indication for removal of native kidneys?	Uncontrollable HTN, ongoing renal sepsis

IMMUNOSUPPRESSION _____

For cadaveric xplant?	Cyclosporine, Imuran, steroids, ATG, OKT3
For LRD xplant?	Cyclosporine, Imuran, steroids

REJECTION _____

Red flag?	Increasing creatinine
Differential for ↑Cr?	(Remember: "**-tion**") obstruc*tion,* dehydra*tion,* infec*tion,* intoxica*tion* (CSA); plus lymphocele, ATN
Signs/symptoms?	Fever, malaise, HTN, ipsilateral leg edema, pain at xplant site, oliguria
Workup	
a. US/Doppler?	Look for fluid collection around kidney, hydronephrosis, flow in vessels
b. Radionuclide scan?	Look at flow and function
c. Biopsy?	Distinguish between rejection and cyclosporine toxicity
Time course for return of normal renal function after transplant?	LRD—3–5 days Cadaveric—7–15 days

LIVER TRANSPLANT

Indications?
Liver failure due to

1. Cirrhosis (#1 in adults)
2. Budd-Chiari
3. Biliary atresia (#1 in children)
4. Neonatal hepatitis
5. Chronic active hepatitis
6. Fulminant hepatitis with drug toxicity—Tylenol
7. Sclerosing cholangitis
8. Caroli's disease
9. Subacute hepatic necrosis
10. Congenital hepatic fibrosis
11. Inborn errors of metabolism
12. Fibrolamellar hepatocellular carcinoma

Define

Liver failure?
Stage III or IV encephalopathy in patient with liver disease, also abnormal synthetic function

Stage III encephalopathy?
Deep somnolence, incoherent speech

Stage IV encephalopathy?
Coma

Tests for compatibility?
ABO typing

Placement?
Orthotopic

Size?
Donor body weight should be approx 50%> or 50%< than recipient

Immunosuppression?
Cyclosporine, Imuran, steroids

REJECTION

Red flags?
Decreased bile drainage, increased serum bilirubin, increased LFTs

Site of rejection?
Rejection involves the biliary epithelium first and later the vascular endothelium

WORKUP OF REJECTION

a. U/S with Doppler?
Look at flow in portal vein, hepatic artery; r/o thrombosis, leaky anastomosis, infection (abscess)

b. Cholangiogram?	Look at bile ducts; easy to do (patients usually have a T-tube if they have 1° biliary anastomosis)
c. Biopsy?	Especially 3–6 weeks postop, when most worried about CMV
Why get renal failure s/p liver transplant?	#1 reason is preop hepatorenal failure (which is reversible with xplant), then intraop hypotension, sepsis, injury, cyclosporine toxicity

SURVIVAL STATISTICS

1-year survival?	About 80%
What percentage of patients require retransplant?	About 20%
Why?	Usually due to primary graft dysfunction, rejection, infection, or vascular thrombosis

PANCREAS TRANSPLANT

Indications?	Type I, juvenile diabetes mellitus but before end-stage bad complications (renal failure, blindness, neuropathy)
Tests for compatibility?	ABO, Dr matching (class II)
Placement?	Heterotopic, in iliac fossa or paratopic
Anastomosis of exocrine duct (in heterotopic)?	To bladder
Why?	Can measure the amount of amylase in urine, gives an indication of pancreatic fxn (i.e., high urine amylase indicates good pancreatic fxn)
Complication?	Loss of bicarbonate
Anastomosis of exocrine duct in paratopic?	To jejunum
Why?	It is close by and it's physiologic
Advantage of paratopic?	Endocrine fxn drains to portal vein directly to liver and pancreatic contents stay within the GI tract—no need to replace bicarb
Immunosuppression?	Cyclosporine, Imuran, steroids
Rejection red flags?	Hyperamylasemia, hyperglycemia, hypoamylasuria, graft tenderness

| Why transplant kidney and pancreas together? | Kidney fxn better indicator of rejection, also better survival of graft for kidney-pancreas than pancreas alone |

HEART TRANSPLANT

Indications?	Age 0–65 with terminal acquired heart disease—class IV of New York Heart Assoc classification (inability to do any physical activity without discomfort = 10% chance of surviving 6 mo)
Contraindications?	Over age 65 (variable) Active infection Poor pulmonary function Increased pulmonary artery resistance
Tests for compatibility?	ABO, size
Placement?	Orthotopic anastomosis of atria, Ao, pulmonary artery
Immunosuppression?	Cyclosporine, Imuran, steroids

REJECTION _____

| Red flags? | Fever, hypo- or hypertension, increased T4/T8 ratio |
| Tests? | Endomyocardial biopsy—much more important than clinical signs/symptoms patient undergoes routine bx |

SURVIVAL STATISTICS _____

| 1-year graft survival? | 85–95% |

LUNG TRANSPLANT

Indications?	Generally, disease that substantially limits activities of daily living and is likely to result in death within 12–18 months
	Pulmonary fibrosis COPD Eosinophilic granuloma Primary pulmonary HTN Eisenmenger's syndrome Cystic fibrosis
Contraindications?	Current smoking Active infection Current steroid therapy

Pretransplant assessment? of recipient?	1. Pulmonary—PFTs, V/Q scan 2. Cardiac—Echo, cath, angiogram 3. Exercise tolerance test
Donor requirements?	1. Age < 55 2. Clear chest film 3. PA oxygen tension of 300 on 100% oxygen and 5 cm PEEP 4. No purulent secretions on bronchoscopy
Necessary anastomoses?	Bronchi, PA, pulmonary veins Bronchial artery not necessary
Red flags of rejection?	1. Decreased arterial O_2 tension 2. Fever 3. Increased fatiguability 4. Infiltrate on x-ray

SURVIVAL STATISTICS _____

Single lung, 1 year?	About 65%
Double lung, 1 year?	About 70%

TRANSPLANT COMPLICATIONS

Note 4 major complications	1. Infection 2. Rejection 3. Posttransplant lymphoma 4. Complications of steroids

INFECTION _____

Usual agents?	DNA viruses, especially CMV, HSV
When begin to suspect CMV infection?	21 days posttransplant
Signs/Sx of CMV?	Clinical illness of fever, neutropenia, signs of rejection of xplant; also can present as viral pneumonitis, hepatitis, colitis
Diagnosis of CMV?	Biopsy of xplant to differentiate rejection, cultures of blood, urine
Treatment of CMV?	Ganciclovir +/− immunoglobin
Complications?	Bone marrow suppression
Signs/Sx of HSV?	Herpetic lesions, shingles, fever, neutropenia, rejection of xplant
Treatment of HSV?	Acyclovir until asymptomatic

MALIGNANCY _____

Most common types?	75% of malignancies that develop are lymphoid or epithelial in origin

Which epithelial cancers are important s/p xplant?

Skin cancer—esp. basal cell, squamous cell and carcinoma in situ of cervix

Treatment of malignancy?

Epithelial—standard operative procedure; lymphomas are difficult to treat and lead to death in most patients

Posttransplant lymphoma is associated with?

Multiple doses of OKT3

44
Orthopaedic Surgery

GENERAL PRINCIPLES

How are fractures described?

1. Type of fx (open or closed)
2. Bone (by thirds: prox/middle/distal)
3. Pattern of fracture, e.g., comminuted
4. Degree of angulation

How do you define the degree of angulation and/or displacement?

Define lateral/medial/anterior/posterior displacement and angulation of the distal fragment(s) in relation to the proximal bone

Define the Following _____

1. Diaphysis

1. Main shaft of long bone

2. Metaphysis

2. Flared end of long bone

3. Physis

3. Growth plate, found only in immature bone

4. Epiphysis

4. End of long bone

Potential fracture sites

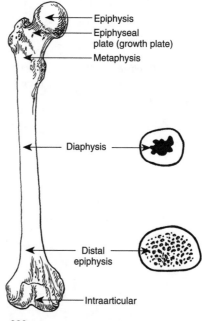

Epiphysis
Epiphyseal plate (growth plate)
Metaphysis

Diaphysis

Distal epiphysis

Intraarticular

FRACTURES

DEFINE THE FOLLOWING PATTERNS OF FRACTURE _____

Closed fracture	Intact skin over fracture/hematoma
Open fracture	Wound overlying fracture, through which fracture fragments are in continuity with outside environment; high risk of infection *Note:* Called compound fracture in past
Simple fracture	1 fracture line, 2 bone fragments
Comminuted fracture	Results in >2 bone fragments; also known as fragmentation

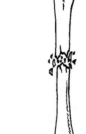

Comminuted fracture

Transverse fracture	Fracture line perpendicular to long axis of bone

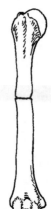

Transverse fracture

Oblique fracture

Fracture line creates an oblique angle w/long axis of bone

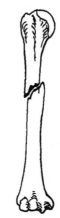

Oblique fracture

Spiral fracture

Severe oblique fracture in which fracture plane rotates along the long axis of bone; caused by a twisting injury

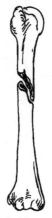

Spiral fracture

Longitudinal fracture

Fracture line parallel to long axis of bone

Impacted fracture

Fracture due to compressive force; end of bone is driven into contiguous metaphyseal region *without* displacement

Pathologic fracture

Fracture through abnormal bone, e.g., tumor-laden or osteoporotic bone

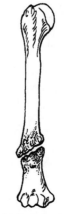

Pathologic fracture

Stress fracture

Fracture in normal bone due to cyclic loading on bone

Greenstick fracture

Incomplete fracture in which cortex on only one side is disrupted; seen in children

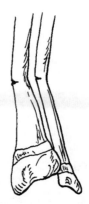

Greenstick fracture

Torus fracture

Impaction injury in children where cortex is buckled but not disrupted (A.K.A. buckle fracture)

Displaced fracture

Occurs when cortices of fractured bone are knocked out of alignment *without* angulation; the *displacement* is measured and noted

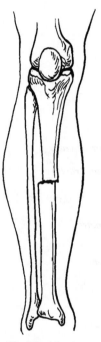

Displaced fracture

Angulated fracture

Occurs when an angle is created b/w the long axes of the two main bone fragments; the *angulation* is measured and noted

Rotated fracture

Occurs when one bone fragment rotates in relation to the other along the longitudinal axis; the rotation is usually difficult to see on x-ray and is usually noted clinically

Avulsion fracture	Fracture in which tendon is pulled from bone, carrying with it a bone chip

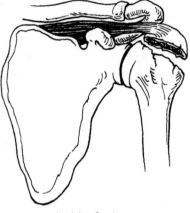

Avulsion fracture

Periarticular fracture	Fracture close to but not involving the joint
Intraarticular fracture	Fracture through the articular surface of a bone

DEFINE THE FOLLOWING SPECIFIC FRACTURES _____

Colles' fracture	Fracture of the distal end of the radius, usually from falling on an outstretched hand
Jones' fracture	Fracture at base of 5th metatarsal diaphysis
Bennet's fracture	Fracture of the base of the first metacarpal with involvement of carpometacarpal joint
Smith's fracture	Opposite of Colles' fx; fracture of distal radius but from falling on the dorsum of the hand
Boxer's fracture	Fracture of the metacarpal neck, "classically" of small finger
Clay shoveler's fracture	Fracture of spinous process of C7
Hangman's fracture	Fracture of the pedicles of C2
Transcervical fracture	Fracture through neck of femur
Monteggia fracture	Fracture of the proximal one-third of the ulna with a dislocation of the radial head
Galeazzi fracture	Fracture of the radius at the junction of the middle and distal thirds accompanied by disruption of the distal radioulnar joint
Pott's fracture	Fracture of distal fibula

Pott's disease	Tuberculosis of the spine

OTHER ORTHOPAEDIC TERMS

Reduction	Maneuver to restore proper alignment to fracture or joint
Closed reduction	Reduction done *without* surgery, e.g., casts, splints
Open reduction	Surgical reduction
Fixation	Stabilization of a fracture after reduction by means of surgical placement of hardware (pins, plates, screws, etc.); can be external or internal
Unstable fracture or dislocation	Fracture or dislocation in which further deformation will occur if reduction is *not* performed
Varus	Extremity abnormality with apex of defect pointed away from midline; e.g., genu varum = bowlegged; with valgus, this term can also be used to describe fracture displacement (think, knees are very VARIED apart)

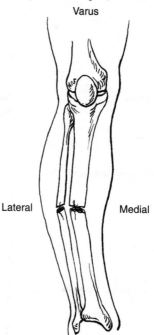

Varus

Lateral   Medial

Valgus

Extremity abnormality w/ apex of defect pointed toward the midline; e.g., genu valgus = knock-kneed

Valgus

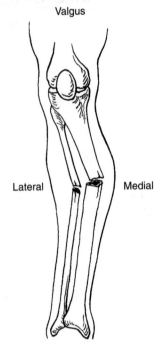

Lateral   Medial

Dislocation

Total loss of congruity b/w articular surfaces of a joint

Subluxation

Anything *less than total* loss of congruity between articular surfaces

ORTHOPAEDIC TRAUMA

What factors determine the *extent of injury?*

1. *Age:* suggests susceptible point in musculoskeletal system:
   Child—growth plate
   Adolescent—ligaments
   Elderly—metaphyseal bone
2. *Direction of forces*
3. *Magnitude of forces*

What are indications for *open reduction?*

1. Intraarticular fractures
2. Extremity function requiring perfect reduction
3. Failed closed reduction

4. Multiple trauma; to allow mobilization at earliest possible date
5. Elderly patients where a long period w/o ambulation carries a risk of compromised cardiopulmonary function

What are the major *orthopaedic emergencies?*

1. Open fractures/dislocations
2. Vascular injuries
3. Compartment syndromes
4. Neural compromise, especially spinal injury
5. Osteomyelitis/septic arthritis; acute, i.e., when aspiration is indicated
6. Hip dislocations—require immediate reduction or patient will develop avascular necrosis; "reduce on the x-ray table"

What is the *main risk* when dealing with an *open fracture*?

Infection

How are open fractures classified?

By amount of tissue injury and bony exposure
  Grade I: <1 cm soft tissue laceration
  Grade II: >1 cm soft tissue laceration with moderate contamination
  Grade III:
    A. Usually >10 cm severe tissue injury with high contamination
    B. III A + need for skin graft for soft tissue coverage
    C. IIIA or B + vascular injury requiring repair

Initial treatment of open fracture?

1. Prophylactic abx to include IV Gram pos and anaerobic coverage
    Grade I—Ancef
    Grade II or III—Cefoxitin + pcn/gent
2. Surgical debridement
3. Inoculation against tetanus
4. Lavage wound <6 hr postincident with high-pressure sterile water
5. Open reduction of fx
6. Stabilization; e.g., use of external fixation

What is *acute compartment syndrome?*

Increased pressure within an osseofascial compartment that leads to compromised circulation and function

What are causes?	Fractures, vascular compromise, reperfusion injury, but can occur after *any* musculoskeletal injury
What situations should immediately alert one to be on the lookout for a developing compartment syndrome?	1. Supracondylar elbow fractures in children 2. Proximal/midshaft tibial fxs 3. Electrical burns 4. Arterial/venous disruption
How is the diagnosis made?	Tight extremity + pressures > 30–40 mm Hg 5 P's: 1. Pain 2. Pallor 3. Pulselessness (not 100%!) 4. Paresthesia 5. Paralysis
Can a patient have a compartment syndrome with a palpable or Doppler-detectable distal pulse?	YES!
What is the Rx?	Fasciotomy within 6–8 hours
What if fx, no pulse, but no compartment syndrome?	Arteriogram
How do peripheral nerve injuries usually occur?	From trauma to extremities
What are the neural concerns in closed injuries?	Nerve exploration usually not indicated because nerves tend to recover alone, but attention should be directed at muscles/joints to prevent contraction and/or stretching
What about in penetrating wounds?	Nerve transection is common; exploratory surgery is often indicated
What are the types of spinal fractures?	1. *Chance fx*—Fracture transverse spinal through vertebrae, often secondary to seatbelt restraint during MVA 2. *Compression fx*—Anterior wedging of vertebrae secondary to axial loading; seen most frequently in elderly with osteoporosis 3. *Burst fx*—Compression of vertebrae both anteriorly and posterior with high force; often with retropulsion of fragments into spinal canal (see Fig. 7)

DISLOCATIONS

SHOULDER

Most common type?	95% are anterior (posterior are often seen with epilepsy or electrocution)
Structures at risk?	Axillary nerve + axillary artery
Dx?	Indentation of soft tissue beneath acromion
Rx?	1. Reduction via gradual traction 2. Immobilize × 3 weeks in internal rotation 3. ROM exercises

ELBOW

Most common type?	Posterior
Structures at risk?	Brachial a
Rx?	Reduce and splint for 7–10 days

HIP

Most common type?	Posterior—"Dashboard dislocation"—often involves fx of posterior lip of acetabulum
Structures at risk?	Sciatic n. Blood supply to femoral head—AVN
Rx?	Closed or open reduction

KNEE

Most common type?	Anterior or posterior
Structures at risk?	Popliteal a. and v., peroneal n.—especially with posterior dislocation *Note:* need arteriogram
Rx?	Often requires ligament repair of reconstruction

COMMON FRACTURES AND DISLOCATIONS IN ADULTS

What is a chief concern in humeral shaft fractures?	Radial nerve palsy
What *must* be done when both forearm bones are broken?	Because precise movements are needed, open reduction and internal fixation are a must.
How have femoral fractures been repaired traditionally?	Traction for 4–6 weeks
Newer technique?	Intramedullary rod placement
Advantages?	Nearly immediate mobility with decreased morbidity/mortality
What is the chief concern following tibial fractures?	Recognition of associated compartment syndrome

When do hip dislocations usually occur?	High-velocity injuries, e.g., MVA
Pain in anatomical snuffbox suggests?	Fracture of scaphoid bone (A.K.A. navicular fx)

ROTATOR CUFF

What muscles form the rotator cuff?	1. *S*upraspinatus (acronym = ''SITS'') 2. *I*nfraspinatus 3. *T*eres minor 4. *S*ubscapularis
When do tears usually occur?	5th decade
What is the usual hx?	Hx of intermittent shoulder pain followed by episode of acute pain corresponding to a tendon tear; weakness of abduction
What is Rx?	1. Most tears: symptomatic pain relief 2. Later: if poor muscular function persists, surgical repair is indicated

DEFINE

1. Volkmann's contracture	Contracture of forearm flexors secondary to **forearm compartment syndrome**
Usual cause?	Brachial artery injury, **supracondylar humerus fx,** radius/ulnar fx, crush injury, etc.
2. Dupuytren's contracture	Thickening + contracture of palmar fascia; incidence increases with age

ORTHOPAEDIC INFECTIONS

OSTEOMYELITIS _____

What is osteomyelitis?	Inflammation/infection of bone marrow and adjacent bone
What are the most likely causative organisms?	*Neonates: Staphylococcus* A, Gram − *Child: Staphylococcus* A, *H. influenzae* *Adults: Staphylococcus* A *Immunocompromised/drug addicts: Gram −* *Sickle cell: Salmonella, Staphylococcus*
What seen on PE?	Tenderness, ↓ movement, swelling
What are Dx steps?	H/P, needle aspirate, CBC, ESR, bone scan
What are Rx options?	Antibiotics +/− surgical drainage

SEPTIC ARTHRITIS _____

What is septic arthritis?	Inflammation of a joint beginning as synovitis and ending with destruction of articular cartilage if left untreated
Causative agents?	Same as in osteomyelitis except gonococcus is #1 in adult population
Physical exam?	Joint pain, ↓ motion, joint swelling, joint warm to touch
Dx steps?	Needle aspirate, look for pus; Culture + Gram stain
Necessary treatment?	Decompression of joint via needle aspiration + IV abx; hip, shoulder, and spine must be surgically incised, debrided, and drained

ORTHOPAEDIC TUMORS

What is the most common type?	*METASTASIS!*
Common sources	Breast, lung, prostate, kidney, and multiple myeloma
Usual presentation	May present as bone pain or as a pathologic fracture
Most common primary malignant bone tumor?	Multiple myeloma
What is the differential diagnosis for a possible bone tumor?	1. Metastatic disease 2. 1° bone tumors 3. Metabolic disorder, e.g., hyperparathyroidism 4. Infection
What are the benign bone tumors?	1. Osteochondroma 2. Enchondroma 3. Unicameral bone cyst 4. Osteoid osteoma 5. Chondroblastoma 6. Fibroxanthoma 7. Fibrous dysplasia
What are the malignant bone tumors?	1. Osteosarcoma 2. Chondrosarcoma 3. Ewing's sarcoma 4. Giant cell tumor (locally malignant) 5. Malignant melanoma 6. Metastatic

What are Dx steps?	1. PE/lab tests
	2. Radiographs
	3. CT and/or technetium scan
	4. Biopsy
What are radiographic signs of malignant tumors?	1. Large size
	2. Aggressive bone destruction
	3. Ineffective bone rxn to tumor
	4. *EXTENSION* to soft tissues
Benign tumor?	1. Small
	2. Well circumscribed
	3. Lytic lesion with sclerotic rim
	4. *NO* extension

What are some specific radiographic findings of the following:

1. Osteosarcoma?	1. "Sunburst pattern"
2. Fibrous dysplasia?	2. Radiolucent, "ground glass"
3. Ewing's sarcoma?	3. "Onion skinning"

What is mainstay of Rx? Surgery (excision + debridement) for both malignant and benign lesions; XRT and chemo as adjuvant for many malignant tumors

OSTEOSARCOMA

Age at presentation?	10–20 years, M > F
Most common location?	≈⅔ in distal femur, proximal tibia
Radiographic sine qua non?	Bone formation somewhere within tumor
What is Rx?	Resection + chemotherapy
Survival, 5 yr?	About 15%
Most common met site?	Lungs

What is the most common benign bone tumor? *Osteochondroma;* it is cartilaginous in origin and may undergo malignant degeneration

What is a chondrosarcoma? Malignant tumor of cartilaginous origin; presents in middle age and older and is unresponsive to chemo and radiotherapy

EWING'S SARCOMA

Presentation?	Pain, swelling in involved area
Most common location?	Around knee (distal femur, proximal tibia)
Age at presentation?	Evenly spread among those <20
Radiographic findings?	Lytic lesion with periosteal reaction termed "onion skinning," which is calcified layering

What is a unicameral bone cyst?	Fluid-filled cyst most commonly found in prox. humerus in children ages 5–15 years
Presentation?	Pain, pathologic fracture
Rx?	Steroid injections

ARTHRITIS

Which arthritides are classified as degenerative?	1. Osteoarthritis 2. Posttraumatic arthritis
What characterizes Osteoarthritis?	1. Heberden's nodes
Posttraumatic arthritis?	2. *Symmetry,* usually of hip, knee, or spine Usually involves *one joint* of past trauma
What are Rx options for degenerative arthritis?	1. NSAIDS for acute flare-ups, *not* for long-term management 2. Local corticosteroid injections 3. Surgery
What characterizes rheumatoid arthritis?	Autoimmune reaction where hyaline articular cartilage is attacked by invasive pannus
What is *pannus?*	Inflammatory exudate overlying synovial cells inside joint
What are Rx options?	1st level: NSAIDS, long-term management 2nd level: Gold, antimalarials 3rd level: Immunosuppressants
Surgical management choices for joint/bone diseases?	1. Arthroplasty 2. Arthrodesis (fusion) 3. Osteotomy

DEFINE _____

Arthroplasty	Total joint replacement; contraindicated in postinfectious arthritis, e.g., hip arthroplasty; limited durability (10–15 yr) so not recommended in younger patients
Arthrodesis	Joint surface is excised and joint immobilized so joint heals in fixed position, thus stable and painless; good choice for younger patients because durable and long-lasting, e.g., hip arthrodesis in young vs. arthroplasty in elderly
Osteotomy	Cutting bone and realigning joint surfaces, e.g., Coventry type where weight-bearing axis of body is changed to lateral condyle of knee

PEDIATRIC ORTHOPAEDICS

CONGENITAL HIP DISLOCATION

Epidemiology? F > M, firstborn, breech presentation

Which side usually affected? Bilateral 10% of time

Diagnosis? *Barlow's test:* ability to cause subluxation of hip when flexed at 90°; examiner feels/listens for click

Ortolani's sign: reduction of subluxation by abduction

Radiographic confirmation: required

Treatment? Pavlik harness—maintains hip reduction with hips flexed at 100–110°

SCOLIOSIS

Definition? Lateral curvature of a portion of the spine

Nonstructural: corrects with positional change

Structural: does not correct

Cause? Most cases are termed idiopathic, but causes may include neuromuscular paralysis, painful lesion, radiation, thoracic surgery, and congenital anomalies.

Classic presentation? Right thoracic curve, though thoracolumbar, lumbar, and double curves are seen; look for chest rotation and rib hump.

Epidemiology? Usually affects prepubertal females

Rx options?
1. Braces
2. Surgery
3. Electrical stimulation

DEFINE

Legg-Calvé-Perthes disease Idiopathic avascular necrosis of femoral head in children

Slipped capital femoral epiphysis Migration of proximal femoral epiphysis of child on the metaphysis

Note: **Hip pain in children often presents as knee pain**

Blount's disease Idiopathic varus bowing of tibia

SALTER CLASSIFICATION

Describes what?	Fractures in children involving physis
Indicates high risk of what?	Growth arrest potential
Define:	
Salter I	Through physeal plate only
Salter II	Involves physis and metaphysis
Salter III	Involves physis and epiphysis
Salter IV	Fracture extends from metaphysis through physis, into epiphysis
Salter V	Axial force crushes physeal plate

SELECTED PEDIATRIC FRACTURES

Why is the growth plate of concern in childhood fxs?

The growth plate represents the "weak link" in the musculoskeletal system of the child. Fractures involving the growth plate of long bones may compromise normal growth, so special attention should be given to them.

What is a chief concern when oblique/spiral fxs of long bones are seen in children?

Child abuse is a possibility and other signs of abuse should be investigated

What is usually done during reduction of a femoral fx?

During reduction a small amount of overlap is allowed because ↑ vascularity due to injury may make the affected limb *longer* if overlap is not present. Treatment after reduction is a spica cast.

What of ligamentous injury in children?

Most "ligamentous" injuries are actually fractures involving the growth plate!

What two fractures have a high incidence of associated compartment syndrome?

1. Tibial fractures
2. Supracondylar fractures of humerus (Volkmann's contracture)

SPINE

LUMBAR DISC HERNIATION _____

Define?

Extrusion of the inner portion of the intervertebral disc (nucleus pulposus) through the outer annulus fibrosis, causing impingement on nerve roots exiting the spinal canal

Which nerve is affected?

The nerve exiting at the level below (e.g., an L4-L5 disc impinges on the L5 nerve exiting between L5-S1)

Who is affected?

Middle-aged and older individuals

Usual cause?

Loss of elasticity of the posterior longitudinal ligaments and annulus fibrosis due to aging

Most common sites?

L5-S1 45%
L4-L5 40%

Presenting symptom?

Usually low back pain

Signs?
  L5-S1?

Decreased ankle jerk reflex
Weakness of plantar flexors in foot
Pain in back/midgluteal region to posterior calf to lateral foot
Ipsilateral radiculopathy on straight leg raise

  L4-L5?

Decreased biceps femoris reflex
Weak extensors of foot
Pain in hip/groin region to posterolateral thigh, lateral leg, and medial toes

Diagnosis?

CT myelogram or MRI

Treatment?

Conservative—bed rest and analgesics
Surgical—hemilaminectomy and discectomy

CERVICAL DISC DISEASE _____

Define?	Basically the same pathology as above, except in the cervical region; the disc impinges on the nerve exiting the canal at the same level of the disease (e.g., a C6-C7 disc impinges on the C7 nerve root exiting at the C6-C7 foramen)
Most common sites?	C6-C7 70% C5-C6 20%
Signs/Sx? **C7?**	Decreased triceps reflex/strength Pain from neck, through triceps and into index and middle finger
C6?	Decreased biceps and brachioradialis reflex Weakness in forearm flexion Pain in neck, radial forearm, and thumb
Spurling's sign?	Reproduction of radicular pain by having the patient turn head to affected side and examiner applying axial pressure to top of head
Diagnosis?	CT or MRI
Treatment?	Same as with lumbar disc disease
Symptoms of central cervical cord compression from disc fragments?	Myelopathic syndrome with LMN signs at level of compression and UMN signs distally; e.g., C7 compression may cause bilateral loss of triceps reflex and bilateral hyperreflexia, clonus, and Babinski signs in lower extremities

SPINAL EPIDURAL ABSCESS _____

Etiology?	Hematogenous spread from skin infections is most common; also, distant abscesses/infections, UTIs, postop infections, and LPs
Commonly associated medical condition?	Diabetes mellitus
Most common sites?	1. Thoracic 2. Lumbar 3. Cervical
Most common organism?	*Staphylococcus aureus*

Signs/Sx?	Fever; severe pain over affected area and with flexion/extension of spine; weakness can develop, ultimately leading to paraplegia
Diagnosis?	MRI is test of choice.
Contraindicated test?	LP because of risk of seeding CSF with bacteria, causing meningitis
Treatment?	Surgical drainage and appropriate antibiotic coverage
Prognosis?	Depends on preop condition; severe neuro deficits (e.g., paraplegia) show little recovery; 15–20% of cases are fatal

SYRINGOMYELIA

Definition?	Central pathologic cavitation of the spinal cord
Etiology?	Unknown, but associated with cranial base malformations, intramedullary tumors, or traumatic necrosis of the cord
Anatomic location?	Most are in cervical/upper thoracic region; they can extend either way (syringobulbia = extension into medulla)
Signs/Sx?	First, bilateral loss of pain and temperature sensation in "cape-like" distribution (lateral spinothalamic tract involvement); enlargement of syrinx will cause further motor and sensory loss
Diagnosis?	MRI will show defect in cord
Treatment?	Surgical (syringosubarachnoid shunt)

VASCULAR NEUROSURGERY

OCCLUSIVE CEREBROVASCULAR DISEASE

Causes of cerebral infarction?	Thrombosis and embolism
Signs/Sx prior to infarction?	Most important are transient ischemic attacks (TIAs), i.e., temporary ischemic insults to the brain that usually signify cerebrovascular pathology; specific symptoms depend on what area of the brain is ischemic.

Artery most often involved? Middle cerebral artery

Treatment? For severe stenosis (>70%) of internal carotid artery, carotid endarterectomy is the most beneficial treatment. If stenosis is mild (<70%) patients are given a trial of 1 gm ASA per day. A patient who continues to have TIAs during treatment is a surgical candidate.

SUBARACHNOID HEMORRHAGE (SAH)

Usual causes? Most cases are due to **trauma;** of nontraumatic SAH, #1 cause is ruptured **Berry aneurysm,** followed by arteriovenous malformations

What is a Berry aneurysm? Saccular outpouching of vessels in the circle of Willis, usually at bifurcations

Usual location for Berry aneurysm? Anterior communicating a. is #1 (30%), followed by posterior communicating a. and middle cerebral a.

What medical disease increases the risk of Berry aneurysms? Polycystic kidney disease and connective tissue disorders (e.g., Marfan's)

What is an AVM? A congenital abnormality of the vasculature with retainment of one or more primitive connections between the arterial and venous circulations; there is a failure to develop the connecting capillary network

Where do they occur? >75% are supratentorial

Signs/Sx of SAH? Classic symptom is "the worst headache of my life." Meningismus is documented by neck pain and positive Kernig's and Brudzinski's signs. Occasionally LOC, vomiting, and CN deficits occur.

Workup of SAH? If SAH is suspected, head CT should be first test ordered to look for subarachnoid blood. LP may show xanthochromic CSF, but is not necessary if CT is definitive. This should be followed by arteriogram to look for aneurysms or AVMs.

Complications of SAH?	1. Brain edema leading to increased ICP 2. Rebleeding (most common in first 24–48 hours posthemorrhage) 3. Vasospasm (peaks 7–11 days after bleeding) of cerebral arteries is the most common cause of morbidity and mortality
Treatment of aneurysm?	Surgical treatment by placing metal clip on aneurysm is the mainstay of therapy. Alternatives include balloon occlusion or coil embolization.
Treatment of AVM?	Many are on the brain surface and are accessible operatively. Preoperative embolization can reduce the size of the AVM. For surgically inaccessible lesions, radiosurgery has been very effective in treating AVMs < 3 cm in diameter

INTRACEREBRAL HEMORRHAGE

Definition?	Bleeding into the brain parenchyma, as opposed to the subarachnoid, subdural, or epidural space
Etiology?	#1 is hypertensive/atherosclerotic disease giving rise to Charcot-Bouchard aneurysms (small tubular aneurysms along smaller terminal arteries); other causes include coagulopathies, AVMs, amyloid angiopathy, tumors, and trauma
Where does it occur?	⅔ occur in the basal ganglia; putamen is the structure most commonly affected
How often does blood spread to ventricular system?	⅔ of cases
Usual presentation?	⅔ present with coma; large putamen bleeding classically presents with contralateral hemiplegia and hemisensory deficits, lateral gaze preference, aphasia, and homonymous hemianopsia
Surgical indications?	Cerebellar hemorrhages must be removed quickly to decrease the risk of tonsillar herniation and death. Large lobar lesions are also commonly removed.
Prognosis?	Poor, especially with ventricular or diencephalon involvement

TRAUMA

Head Trauma

Incidence?

70,000 fatal injuries/yr in U.S.

What is the Glasgow Coma Scale and why is it important?

The GCS is a measure of brain dysfunction and is used as a predictor of prognosis in head-injured patients. Responses are graded for verbal, motor, and ocular responses. Patients with a GCS score of 3–8 are defined as comatose. Patients with an initial score of 3–4 have a >95% incidence of death or persistent vegetative state.

GCS scoring system
  Eyes?

Eye opening (E)
4—opens spontaneously
3—opens to voice (command)
2—opens to painful stimulus
1—does not open eyes
(Think = "4 eyes")

  Motor?

Motor Response (M)
6—obeys commands
5—localizes painful stimulus
4—withdraws from pain
3—decorticate posture
2—decerebrate posture
1—no movement
(Think = 6-cylinder motor")

  Verbal?

Verbal Response (V)
5—appropriate and oriented
4—confused
3—inappropriate words
2—incomprehensible sounds
1—no sounds

Unilateral, dilated, nonreactive pupil suggests?

Focal mass lesion (e.g., epidural hematoma)

Bilateral fixed and dilated pupils suggest?

Diffusely increased ICP

4 signs of basilar skull fracture?

1. **Raccoon eyes**—periorbital ecchymoses
2. **Battle's sign**—postauricular ecchymoses
3. **Hemotympanum**
4. **CSF** rhinorrhea/otorrhea

Initial radiographic imaging in trauma?

1. Plain films of C-spine (C1-C7)
2. Head CT (esp. if LOC)
3. Other plain films/CT as indicated by exam

What is normal ICP?	5–15 mm H_2O
Worrisome ICP?	>20 mm H_2O
What is Cushing's triad?	Physiologic response to increased ICP (A.K.A. Cushing's response)

1. Increased vascular resistance (increasing BP)
2. Bradycardia
3. Respiratory irregularity

General indications to monitor ICP after trauma?

1. GCS < 11–12
2. Altered level of consciousness or unconsciousness with multiple system trauma
3. Decreased consciousness with focal neuro exam abnormality

Nonoperative techniques to decrease ICP?

1. Reverse Trendelenburg position
2. Mannitol (osmotic diuretic)
3. Intubation + hyperventilation
4. Reversible sedation
5. Pharmacologic paralysis
6. Pentobarbital coma (last resort)

How does cranial nerve exam localize the injury in a comatose patient?

The CNs proceed caudally in the brainstem as numbered. Presence of corneal reflex (CN 5 + 7) indicates intact pons. Intact gag reflex (CN 9 + 10) shows functioning upper medulla. Be aware that CN 6 palsy is often a false localizing sign.

What is an epidural hematoma?

Collection of blood between the calvaria and dura

What causes it?

Usually occurs in association with a skull fracture as bone fragments lacerate meningeal arteries

What artery is associated with epidural hematomas?

Middle meningeal artery

Cause of subdural hematomas?

Tearing of veins that pass through the space between the cortical surface and the dural venous sinuses or injury to the brain surface with resultant bleeding from cortical vessels

3 Types of subdurals?

1. Acute—symptoms within 72 hr of injury
2. Subacute—3–20 days
3. Chronic—3 weeks or longer

Treatment of epidural and subdural hematomas?	The mass effect (pressure) must be reduced. While the medical measures mentioned above can be employed to delay additional neurologic damage, craniotomy with the removal of clot is required. The surgeon must address any remaining bleeding to prevent reaccumulation of the hematoma.
What is a depressed skull fracture?	A fracture in which one or more fragments of the calvarium is forced below the inner table of the skull.
Surgical indications?	1. Contaminated wound requiring cleaning and debridement 2. Cosmetic purposes (esp. frontal bone) 3. Impingement on cortex

SPINAL CORD TRAUMA

2 General types of injury?	1. Complete: no motor/sensory function below the level of injury 2. Incomplete: residual function below level of injury

Describe

Anterior cord syndrome?	**Anterior cord syndrome**—affects corticospinal and lateral spinothalamic tracts, paraplegia, loss of pain/temp sensation
Central cord syndrome?	**Central cord syndrome**—preservaton of some lower extremity motor and sensory ability
Brown-Séquard Syndrome?	**Brown-Séquard syndrome**—hemisection of cord resulting in ipsilateral motor weakness and touch/proprioception loss with contralateral pain/temperature loss
Posterior cord syndrome?	Posterior cord syndrome—injury to posterior spinal cord with loss of proprioception distally
Important initial labs/ intervention?	1. ABCs—obtain airway and vent if needed 2. Maintain BP 3. NG tube—prevents aspiration 4. Foley—bladder incontinence 5. High-dose steroids—proven to improve outcome 6. Complete cervical x-rays and those of lower levels as indicated by exam

Define

Jefferson's fracture?	Fracture through **C1** arches due to axial loading (unstable fracture)

Hangman's fracture?	Fracture through the pedicles of **C2** due to hyperextension. Usually stable. Think: hangman (C2) is below stature of President T. Jefferson (C1)
Odontoid fracture?	Fracture of the odontoid process of C2. (view with open-mouth odontoid x-ray)
Priapism?	Penile erection seen with spinal cord injury

TUMORS

GENERAL

Incidence of CNS tumors?	1% of all cancer; 3rd leading cause of cancer deaths in people 15–34; 2nd leading cause of cancer deaths in children
Define benign vs. malignant in the setting of CNS tumors	Malignant tumors are highly aggressive/proliferative tumors of poorly differentiated cells. Benign refers to a less aggressive, more differentiated cell line. However, a benign tumor can be as lethal as a malignant variety because of the continued ability to grow within the confines of the skull.
Usual location of primary tumors in adults/children?	In adults, roughly ⅔ of tumors are supratentorial, ⅓ infratentorial. The reverse is true in children.
Adverse effects of tumors on the brain?	1. Increased ICP 2. Mass effect on cranial nerves 3. Invasion of brain parenchyma, disrupting nuclei/tracts 4. Seizure foci 5. Hemorrhage into/around the tumor mass
Signs/Sx of brain tumors?	1. Neuro deficit ⅔ 2. Headache ½ 3. Seizures ¼ 4. Vomiting
Diagnosis?	CT or MRI with and without contrast is the standard diagnostic study.
Surgical indications?	1. Establishing a tissue diagnosis 2. Relief of increased ICP 3. Relief of neurologic dysfunction due to tissue compression 4. Attempt to cure in setting of localized tumor

| Most common intracranial tumors in adults? | Metastatic neoplasm is most common; among primaries, gliomas are #1 ($\frac{1}{2}$) and meningiomas #2 ($\frac{1}{4}$) |
| In children? | 1. Medulloblastomas $\frac{1}{3}$
2. Astrocytomas $\frac{1}{3}$
3. Ependymomas (10%) |

GLIOMAS

What is a glioma?	''Glioma'' is a general name for a number of tumors from neural origin (e.g., astrocytes, oligodendrocytes) which show a wide range of presentations.
Most common glioma?	**Astrocytoma** ($\frac{1}{2}$ of all gliomas)
Most common primary brain tumor in adults?	**Glioblastoma multiforme** (GBM)
Characteristics?	Poorly defined, highly aggressive tumors occurring in the white matter of the cerebral hemispheres; they spread extremely rapidly
Average age of onset?	5th decade
Treatment?	Surgical debulking followed by radiation therapy
Prognosis?	Without treatment, >90% die within 3 months of diagnosis. With treatment, 90% are dead within 2 years

MENINGIOMAS

Peak age of occurrence?	40–50
Sex ratio?	Females predominate almost 2:1
Clinical presentation?	Variable depending on location; lateral cerebral convexity tumors can cause focal deficits or headache; sphenoid tumors can present with seizures; posterior fossa tumors with CN deficits; olfactory groove tumors with anosmia
Treatment?	Surgical resection is the treatment of choice and is usually aimed at complete removal of the tumor.

CEREBELLAR ASTROCYTOMAS

| Peak age of occurrence? | 5–9 years |
| Usual location? | Usually in the cerebellar hemispheres, less frequently in the vermis |

Signs/Sx?	Usually lateral cerebellar signs occur: ipsilateral incoordination or dysmetria (patient tends to fall to side of tumor), as well as nystagmus and ataxia; CN deficits are also frequently present, esp. CNs VI and VII
Treatment and prognosis?	Completely resectable in ¾ of cases which usually results in a cure; overall 5-year survival exceeds 90%

MEDULLOBLASTOMA

Peak age of occurrence?	1st decade
Most common location?	Cerebellar vermis in children; cerebellar hemispheres of adolescents and adults
Signs/Sx?	Headache, vomiting, and other signs of increased ICP; also usually truncal ataxia
Treatment and prognosis?	Best current treatment includes surgery to debulk the tumor, cranial and spinal radiation, and chemotherapy; 5-year survival = ⅔

METASTATIC TUMORS

What are the three main patterns of intracranial metastasis and what are the most common primary tumors involved?	Metastases to 1. Skull/dura: breast, prostate, multiple myeloma 2. Brain parenchyma: lung, breast, skin, kidney, GI tract 3. Meningeal carcinomatosis: lung, leukemia, lymphoma, breast, GI
Where do cerebral mets occur within the brain?	At junction of gray and white matter
Signs/Sx?	Elevated ICP signs, seizures, and focal neurologic deficits; may be abrupt onset or worsening of symptoms with spontaneous hemorrhage into the tumor, which happens more commonly with malignant melanoma, choriocarcinoma, and renal cell carcinoma
Treatment and prognosis?	Surgical resection if lesion is solitary and accessible; otherwise, radiation is most frequently used. Chemo has been used with some success for lung, breast, and testicular primaries. Average survival is about 6 months.

Signs/Sx of meningeal carcinomatosis?	Headache, backache, mental status changes, radiculopathy, and CN palsies are common.
Diagnosis?	Head CT is usually normal, but may show a diffuse enhancement of the meninges. A demonstration of malignant cells in the CSF is required for diagnosis.
Treatment/prognosis?	Intrathecal chemotherapy and radiation; mean survival is about 6 months

PEDIATRIC NEUROSURGERY

HYDROCEPHALUS _____

What is it?	Abnormal condition consisting of an increase in the volume of CSF along with distension of CSF spaces
3 general causes?	1. Increased production of CSF 2. Decreased absorption of CSF 3. Obstruction of flow of normal CSF (90% of cases)
Normal daily CSF production?	≈500 ml
Normal volume of CSF?	≈150 ml in the average adult
Define "communicating" vs. "noncommunicating" hydrocephalus	Communicating: unimpaired connection of CSF pathway from lateral ventricle to subarachnoid space Noncommunicating: Complete or incomplete obstruction of CSF flow within or at the exit of the ventricular system

Specific causes of hydrocephalus?	1. Congenital malformation
	    Aqueductal stenosis
	    Myelomeningocele
	2. Tumors obstructing CSF flow
	3. Inflammation causing impaired absorption of fluid
	    Subarachnoid hemorrhage
	    Meningitis
	4. Choroid plexus papilloma causing increased production of CSF

Signs/Sx?	Signs of increased ICP: HA, nausea, vomiting, ataxia, increasing head circumference exceeding norms for age-related children

Diagnosis?	CT, MRI, measure head circumference
Treatment?	1. Remove obvious offenders 2. Bypass obstruction with ventriculoperitoneal shunt
Prognosis if untreated?	50% mortality; survivors show decreased IQ (mean = 69); neurologic sequelae: ataxia, paraparesis, visual deficits
Complications of treatment?	1. Blockage/shunt malfunction 2. Infection
What is "hydrocephalus ex vacuo"?	Increased volume of CSF spaces due to brain atrophy, not due to any pathology in the amount of CSF absorbed or produced
What is a "shunt series"?	**A series of x-rays covering the entire shunt length—looking for shunt disruption/kinking to explain malfunction of shunt**

Spinal Dysraphism/Neural Tube Defects

Incidence?	Approximately 1/1000 live births in U.S.
Race/gender demographics?	More common in Caucasians and females
Define "spina bifida occulta"	Defect in the development of the posterior portion of the vertebrae
Signs/Sx?	Usually asymptomatic, though it may be associated with other spinal abnormalities; usually found incidentally on x-rays
Most common clinically significant defect?	Myelomeningocele: herniation of nerve roots and spinal cord through a defect in the posterior elements of the vertebra(e); the sac surrounding the neural tissue may be intact, but more commonly is ruptured and therefore exposes the CNS to the external environment
Most common anatomic site?	Lumbar region; next most common is the lower thoracic and upper sacral region
Signs/Sx?	Variable from mild skeletal deformities to a complete motor/sensory loss; bowel/bladder function is difficult to evaluate, but often is affected and can adversely affect survival
Treatment?	With open myelomeningoceles, patients are operated on immediately to prevent infection.

Prognosis?	≈95% survival for first 2 years compared with ¼ in patients not undergoing surgical procedures
Vitamin thought to lower rate of neural tube defects in utero?	Folic acid

CRANIOSYNOSTOSIS

What is it?	Premature closure of one or more of the sutures between the skull plates
Incidence?	1/200 live births in the U.S.
Types?	Named for the suture that is fused (e.g., sagittal, coronal, lambdoid); sagittal craniosynostosis accounts for >50% of all cases; more than one suture can be fused, and all or part of a suture may be affected
Diagnosis?	Physical exam can reveal ridges along fused sutures and lessened suture mobility. Plain x-rays can show a lack of lucency along the fused suture, but are rarely required.
Indications for surgery?	Most often the reasons are cosmetic, as the cranial vault will continue to deform with growth. Occasionally, a child will present with increased ICP secondary to restricted brain growth.
Timing of surgery?	Usually 3–4 months of age; earlier surgery increases the risk of anesthesia; later surgeries are more difficult due to the worsening deformities and decreasing malleability of the skull
Operative mortality?	Less than 1%

MISCELLANEOUS

What anesthetic decreases the seizure threshold?	Enflurane, so **isoflurane** is preferred in neurosurgical cases
Which IV anesthetic causes an increase in ICP?	**Ketamine;** consequently, this medication should be avoided in head trauma patients
Most common cause of postneurosurgery meningitis?	*Staphylococcus aureus* (skin flora)

46
Urology

RENAL CELL CARCINOMA

What is it?

Most common solid renal tumor (90%), also known as hypernephroma, renal adenocarcinoma; originates from proximal renal tubular epithelium

Epidemiology?

Primarily a tumor of adults 40–60 y.o. with 2:1 male to female ratio; makes up <5% of CA in adults; equivalent between whites and blacks

Sx?

Pain (40%), hematuria (35%), wgt loss (35%), flank mass (25%), HTN (20%); classic triad is flank pain, hematuria, and palpable mass; occurs in 10–15%

Dx?

1. IVU
2. U/S to distinguish from benign cyst
3. Abdominal CT with contrast

Staging?

I: Intact renal capsule
II: Extends to perinephric fat
III: (A)IVC or main renal vein
    (B)regional lymph nodes
    (C)vessels and nodes
IV: Distant mets

Metastatic workup?

CXR, IVP, CT, LFTs, serum calcium, bone scan

Sites of mets?

Lung, liver, brain, bone; tumor thrombus entering renal vein or IVC is not uncommon

Treatment?

Radical nephrectomy (excision of the kidney and adrenal including Gerota's fascia) for stages I–IV

BLADDER CANCER

Incidence?

2nd most common urologic malignancy
Male to female ratio of 3:1
Whites > blacks

Histology?	90% transitional cell carcinoma (TCC); remaining are squamous or adeno CA
Risk factors?	Smoking, industrial carcinogens, schistosomiasis
Sx?	Hematuria, irritative sx (frequency, urgency, dysuria)
Workup?	Urinalysis and culture, IVP, cystoscopy with cytology and biopsy
Staging?	O: superficial, limited to mucosa; also known as carcinoma in situ (CIS) A: involves lamina propria B: muscle invasion C: extends to perivesicular fat D: abd organs, lymph nodes
Rx?	Stage O,A: TURB with cautery or laser Recurrent Stages O,A: TURB plus intravesical chemo(BCG, thiotepa) Stages B,C: radical cystectomy Stage D: chemo with irradiation or surgery
What is TURB?	*T*rans-*u*rethral *r*esection of the *b*ladder
Recurrence?	Increased risk b/c of "field effect"; field effect refers to the uniform exposure of the urothelium as it is bathed in urinary carcinogens; Therefore requires surveillance with repeat cystoscopy and urinary cytology every 3–4 months

PROSTATE CANCER

Incidence?	# 1 GU cancer (>100,000 new cases per year in U.S.); most common carcinoma in males in U.S.; 2nd most common cause of death in males in U.S.
Epidemiology?	"A disease of elderly men" present in ⅓ of men age 70–79 and ⅔ aged 80–89 at autopsy; black patients have 50% higher incidence than white patients
Histology?	Adenocarcinoma (95%)
Sx?	Often asymptomatic; usually presents as nodule found on routine rectal exam; in 70% of cases, CA begins in periphery of gland and moves centrally thus obstructive sx come late; 40% have metastatic disease at presentation with sx of bone pain and weight loss

Lymphatic drainage?	Obturator and hypogastric nodes
Common sites of metastasis?	Osteoblastic bony lesions, lung, liver, adrenal
What is the significance of Batson's plexus?	Spinal cord venous plexus; route of isolated skull/brain mets
Early detection and surveillance?	1. Prostate specific antigen (PSA)*—most sensitive and specific marker 2. Acid phosphatase*—often elevated in metastatic prostate CA *used mostly to detect recurrences 3. RECTAL EXAM
Gleason grading system	*Gleason score* 2–4 Well differentiated CA 5–7 Moderately differentiated CA 8–10 Poorly differentiated CA
Dx?	1. Transrectal biopsy 2. Fine needle aspiration
Staging workup?	1. Digital rectal exam 2. Transrectal ultrasonography 3. CT for lymph node involvement 4. Pelvic lymphadenectomy (PLND)—most accurate technique for detecting lymph node involvement 5. PSA 6. Bone scan
Staging?	A: Nonpalpable—confined to prostate B: Palpable nodule, but confined to prostate C: Extends beyond capsule w/o mets D: Metastatic disease

Rx options?
  complications?
	Stage A or B
	1. Radical prostatectomy
	    Leaves 10–50% impotent, depending on age
	    1–10% have incontinence
	2. External beam radiation
	    Intestinal sequelae 5–21%
	    Impotence 22–84%
	Stage C
	Radiation Rx is recommended due to poor results with surgery (disease-free survival is 63/43% at 5/10 years)

Stage D

1. Chemical castration = hormonal tx (palliative); androgen blockade with estrogen Diethylstilbestrol (DES) or LH-RH agonists

2. Surgical castration = orchiectomy (palliative)

Prognosis?	5-year DFS	10 year-DFS
Stage A—surgery	90%	85%
radiation	80%	65%
Stage B—surgery	85%	70%
radiation	70%	50%
Stage C—surgery	60%	45%
radiation	50%	35%

*DFS = Disease-free survival

TESTICULAR CANCER

Incidence?

Rare; 2–3 new cases per 100,000 males per year in U.S.; most common solid tumor of young adult men (20–40 y.o.)

Risk factors?

Cryptorchidism (6% of testicular tumors develop in patients with hx of cryptorchidism)
Relative risk of malignancy
  intraabdominal testis: 1 in 20
  inguinal testis: 1 in 80
Orchiopexy (placement of cryptorchid testis in scrotum) does not alter malignant potential

Sx?

Most present with painless lump, swelling, or firmness of testicle; often noticed after incidental trauma to groin; 10% present with sx of metastatic disease (backpain, anorexia)

Classification?

95% are germ cell tumors
  Seminomatous (35%)
  Nonseminomatous (65%)
    Seminoma (35%)
    Embryonal cell carcinoma (20%)
    Teratoma (5%)
    Mixed cell (40%)
    Choriocarcinoma (<1%)
5% are nongerminal
  Leydig cell
  Sertoli cell
  Gonadoblastoma

Tumor markers?	*HCG*—increased in choriocarcinoma, embryonal carcinoma, and pure seminomas *AFP*—increased in embryonal carcinoma and yolk sac tumors
Workup?	PE, scrotal ultrasound, check tumor markers, CXR, CT
Staging?	
A?	A: confined to testis
B?	B: regional lymph node spread
C?	C: spread beyond retroperitoneal nodes

Rx?	Seminomatous
	    Stages I, IIA: inguinal orchiectomy and RT
	    Stages IIB, III: chemo
	Nonseminomatous:
	    Low stage: orchiectomy and retroperitoneal lymph node dissection (RPLND)
	    High stage: orchiectomy and chemo

What type is most radiosensitive?	**Seminoma;** 95% of stage A can be cured with orchiectomy + radiation (think *S*eminoma = *S*ensitive to radiation)
Why not remove testis with cancer through a scrotal incision?	This could result in tumor seeding of the scrotum
Prognosis?	Excellent for seminomatous and nonseminomatous germ cell tumors in early stages

CALCULUS DISEASE

Incidence?	1 in 10 will have stones
Risk factors?	Poor fluid intake, IBD, hypercalcemia (HPTH, sarcoid), renal tubular acidosis, small bowel bypass
Types of stones?	1. *Calcium oxalate/calcium PO_4*—(75%) secondary to hypercalciuria (increased intestinal absorption, dec. renal reabsorption, increased bone reabsorption) 2. *Struvite (MgAmPh)*—(15%) infection stones; E > M; seen in UTI with urea-splitting bacteria (*Proteus*); may cause staghorn calculi; high urine pH

3. *Uric acid*—(10%) stones are radiolucent; seen in gout, Lesch-Nyhan, chronic diarrhea, CA; low urine pH
4. *Cystine*—(1%) genetic predisposition; radiolucent

What stones are seen in IBD/ bowel bypass?

Calcium oxalate

Sx?

Severe pain! Patient can't sit still; Renal colic (typically pain in kidney/ureter which radiates to testis or penis), hematuria; (remember, patients with peritoneal signs are motionless)

Dx?

KUB (90% radiopaque), IVP, urinalysis and culture, BUN/Cr, CBC

Rx?

Narcotics for pain, vigorous hydration then ESWL (lithotripsy), ureteroscopy, percutaneous litho., open surgery; metabolic workup for recurrence

Indications for intervention?

1. Urinary obstruction
2. Persistent infection
3. Uncontrollable pain
4. Impaired renal function

3 sites of obstruction?

1. Ureteropelvic junction (UPJ)
2. Ureterovesicular junction (UVJ)
3. Where ureter crosses iliac vessels

Prevention?

Increase urine volume
Ca—reduce Ca/oxalate load in diet, tx underlying dz
Struvite—Rx underlying infection
Uric acid—decrease meat in diet, increase pH, allopurinol
Cystine—decrease meat, increase pH, chelaters

INCONTINENCE

Types of incontinence?

1. *True incontinence (TI)*—constant or periodic loss of urine w/o warning, caused by sphincter abn. (exstrophy of bladder)
2. *Stress incontinence (SI)*—loss of urine assoc. with coughing, lifting, exercise, etc.; seen most in women, secondary to relax of pelvic floor following multiple deliveries

3. *Overflow incontinence (OI)*—failure of bladder to empty properly; may be caused by bladder outlet obx (BPH or stricture) or detrusor hypotonicity

4. *Urge incontinence (UI)*—loss of urine secondary to detrusor instability in patient with stroke, dementia, or Parkinson's, etc.

5. *Enuresis*—bedwetting in children

Dx? Hx (including meds), PE (including pelvic/rectal exam), UA, PVR (postvoid residual), urodynamics, cystoscopy / VCUG (*v*esico*c*ysto*u*rethrogram) may be necessary

Rx? *SI*—bladder neck suspension, pessaries, estrogen tx, α-adrenergic stimulation
UI—pharmacotherapy (anticholinergics, α-agonists) bladder denervation, and augmentation cystoplasty
OI—self-cath, surgical relief of obx; avoid using indwelling catheters! (UTIs)
TI—appropriate surgical intervention

BENIGN PROSTATIC HYPERPLASIA

What is it? Dz of elderly men (avg age 60–65 y.o.); prostate gradually enlarges creating sx of urinary outflow obx

Size of normal prostate? 20–25 gm

Where does it occur? BPH occurs periurethrally; prostate CA occurs in periphery of gland

Sx? Obstructive type symptoms: hesitancy, weak stream, nocturia, intermittency, UTI

Dx? History of above sx, digital rectal exam, elevated postvoid residual, U/A, cystoscopy, ultrasound

DDx? Prostate CA—hard gland ... Bx!
Neurogenic bladder—H/O neuro Dz
Acute prostatitis—hot, tender gland
Urethral stricture—retrograde urethrogram, H/O STD

Treatment options? Pharmacologic—α-1 blockade
Hormonal—antiandrogens
Surgical—TURP, TUIP, open prostatectomy
Transurethral balloon dilation

Indications for surgery?	1. Urinary retention 2. Hydronephrosis 3. Recurrent UTIs 4. Bladder stones 5. Severe obstructive Sx
What is "TURP"?	Transurethral resection of prostate

"TUIP"?
  Complications?
	Transurethral incision of prostate
	Immediate: Failure to void
	          Bleeding
	          Clot retention
	          UTI
	Late: Impotence
	    Incontinence
	    Bladder neck contractures

UTI

Etiology?	Ascending infection, instrumentation, sex in females
Common organisms?	1. *E. coli* ≈90% 2. *Proteus* 3. *Klebsiella, Pseudomonas*
Predisposing factors?	Stones, obx, Reflux, DM, pregnancy, indwelling catheter/stent
Sx?	Lower UTI—freq., urgency, dysuria, nocturia Upper UTI—back/flank pain, fever, chills
Dx?	Sx, UA >5 WBCs/hpf, >10^5 CFU grown from clean-catch urine or >10^2 CFU from I and O cath
When to work up?	After first in any **male** (unless Foley in place) After first pyelonephritis in prepubescent female
Rx?	Lower: 1–4 days oral abx Upper: 3–7 days IV abx

WARD QUESTIONS

Does orchiopexy reduce the incidence of testicular neoplasms in undescended testis?	No

Why perform orchiopexy?	1. Decrease the susceptibility to blunt trauma 2. Increase the ease of f/u exams
BPH arises in which area of the prostate?	Periurethral
Prostate CA arises in which area of the prostate?	Periphery
What type of bony lesions do you get from metastatic prostate CA?	Osteo*blastic* (radiopaque)
What percentage of renal cell carcinoma shows evidence of metastatic disease at presentation?	33%
What is the most common site of distant metastasis in RCC?	Lung
What is the most common solid renal tumor of childhood?	Wilms' tumor
What type of renal stone is *radiolucent?*	Uric acid
What are posterior urethal valves?	The most common obstructive urethral lesio: in infants and newborns; occurs only in males; found at distal prostatic urethra
What is the most common intraoperative bladder tumor?	A Foley catheter—don't fall victim!

47
Ophthalmology

GLAUCOMA

What is it?

An ocular disease complex primarily characterized by an **increased intraocular pressure**

What types are there?

1. *Chronic open angle:* bilateral, insidious, slowly progressive; most common type (90%)
2. *Narrow angle:* acute obstruction of aqueous outflow; painful, **acute** visual loss, cloudy cornea
3. *Congenital:* genetically transmitted; often appearing in first year of life

Pathophysiology?

Increased ocular pressure related to increased intraocular aqueous humor production and/or decreased outflow of aqueous humor from the eye, leading to optic nerve degeneration

Diagnosis?

1. Increased intraocular pressure
2. Retinoscopy (optic disc cupping)
3. Peripheral visual field testing

Treatment?

Treatment involves decreasing intraocular pressure through topical eye drops and/or surgery

DIABETIC RETINOPATHY

What is it?

A progressive microangiopathy of retinal blood vessels in diabetic patients

What types are there?

1. *Preproliferative:* retinoscopic hemorrhages *without* neovascularization (precursor of proliferative retinopathy)
2. *Proliferative:* advanced retinoscopic vascular changes *with* neovascularization

Symptoms?

Decreased visual acuity

Diagnosis?

1. Retinoscopy
2. Fluorescein angiogram

339

Treatment?	1. Preproliferative: monitoring for s/s of proliferative retinopathy, blood sugar control
	2. Proliferative: retinal photocoagulation with **argon laser** to peripheral retina

CORNEA

What is keratitis?	Inflammation of the **cornea** secondary to an infectious or mechanical etiology
What infectious agents are frequently involved?	*Staphylococcus, Streptococcus, Pseudomonas,* Herpes, *Chlamydia*
What predisposes the cornea to infection?	Exposure, trauma
Treatment for corneal opacities secondary to scarring?	Corneal transplant
Signs/Sx of corneal abrasions?	Pain! hx of ocular trauma
Dx corneal abrasions?	Fluorescein test

THE RED EYE

What are the eight signs of serious ocular pathology in a red eye?	1. Visual loss
	2. Pain
	3. Opacities
	4. Pupil irregularities
	5. Perilimbal erythema
	6. Increased pressure
	7. History of eye disease
	8. Refractory to treatment

DIFFERENTIAL DIAGNOSIS	*DIAGNOSTIC CLUE:*
Conjunctivitis	**Bacterial:** conjunctival redness with purulent discharge
	Viral: conjunctival redness with serous discharge
	Allergic: conjunctival discharge with clear discharge
Acute narrow angle glaucoma (congenital glaucoma)	Acute pain, cloudy cornea, perilimbal redness, blurred vision
Iritis	Perilimbal redness, irregular pupil, pain, decreased vision

Corneal ulcer	Epithelial defect with infiltrate, pain
Abrasion	Epithelial defect, no infiltrate, pain
Orbital cellulitis	Periocular swelling, erythematous ocular surface, decreased vision

OPHTHALMOLOGY QUESTIONS

What is a cataract?	Opacification of the lens, Tx: surgical removal
What is strabismus?	Misalignment of the eyes
Why is it important to correct strabismus?	To allow proper development of visual acuity and binocular vision
What is a retinal detachment?	A **separation** of the neurosensory retina from the pigment epithelium and its supportive choroid, resulting in retinal infarction
What causes retinal detachment?	Age, trauma, ocular surgery, diabetes—small rent in retina allows fluid to insinuate itself in the subretinal space causing a retinal detachment
What are the signs and Sx of a retinal detachment?	Floaters, blind spots, flashing lights
What is the treatment for a retinal detachment?	Surgery—sclera buckling therapy
What is a pterygium?	A plaque-like extension of fibrovascular tissue onto the cornea
When to remove a blind eye?	Blind and painful, malignancy, blind traumatized eye, diagnostic purposes

DEFINE

Esotropia?	Eyes inward
Exotropia?	Eyes outward
Hypertropia?	Eyes upward
Hypotropia?	Eyes downward
Diplopia?	Double vision
Strabismus?	Eye malalignment
Hyphema?	Blood in anterior chamber of eye

| How does one Rx acid and alkali chemical eye burns? | COPIOUS EYE **IRRIGATION** FOR BOTH! |

What is sympathetic ophthalmia?

Autoimmune destruction of the contralateral **good eye** after penetrating injury causing blindness to ipsilateral eye; remove blind eye before 2 weeks post penetrating injury

Index

Page numbers in italics denote figures.